# `Anyone Who Tells You Vaccines Are Safe And Effective Is Lying. Here's The Proof.'

## Dr Vernon Coleman MB ChB DSc FRSA

**Vernon Coleman: What the papers say:**

`Vernon Coleman writes brilliant books.' - *The Good Book Guide*
`No thinking person can ignore him.' - *The Ecologist*
`The calmest voice of reason.' - *The Observer*
`A godsend.' - *Daily Telegraph*
`Superstar.' - *Independent on Sunday*
`Brilliant!' - *The People*
`Compulsive reading.' - *The Guardian*
`His message is important.' - *The Economist*
`He's the Lone Ranger, Robin Hood and the Equalizer rolled into one.' - *Glasgow Evening Times*
`The man is a national treasure.' - *What Doctors Don't Tell You*
`His advice is optimistic and enthusiastic.' - *British Medical Journal*
`Revered guru of medicine.' - *Nursing Times*
`Hard hitting...inimitably forthright.' - *Hull Daily Mail*
`Refreshingly forthright.' - *Liverpool Daily Post*
`It's impossible not to be impressed.' - *Western Daily Press*
`Outspoken and alert.' - *Sunday Express*
`Controversial and devastating.' - *Publishing News*
`Dr Coleman made me think again.' - *BBC World Service*
`Marvellously succinct, refreshingly sensible.' - *The Spectator*
`Probably one of the most brilliant men alive today.' - *Irish Times*
`King of the media docs.' - *The Independent*
`Britain's leading medical author.' - *The Star*
`Britain's leading health care campaigner.' - *The Sun*
`Perhaps the best known health writer for the general public in the world today.' - *The Therapist*
`The patient's champion.' - *Birmingham Post*
`A persuasive writer whose arguments, based on research and experience, are sound.' - *Nursing Standard*
`The doctor who dares to speak his mind.' - *Oxford Mail*
`He writes lucidly and wittily.' - *Good Housekeeping*

## Note

This book is intended solely to provide information about vaccination. Before contemplating any vaccination you should ask your doctor to confirm that the procedure will be safe and effective for you.

## Dedication

I dedicate this exploration of suppressed and hidden truths to my beloved and beautiful Donna Antoinette who knows, only too well, the heart-wrenching price which must be paid to satisfy the demands of a rapacious industry which is supported by a profession now better known for closed minds and hungry wallets than a dedication to learning and caring.

'We all know there are two sides to every question. There are two sides to a piece of flypaper, too, but it makes a great difference to the fly which side he lands on.' - Peter Seeger

## Preface

Almost everyone who promotes vaccination is paid to do so. The supporters of vaccination have a personal interest in promoting vaccination. On the other hand, just about everyone who questions vaccination does so at great personal cost. Vaccination is big business and many of those who promote it, and make money out of it, do everything they can to protect an intellectually vulnerable but enormously profitable exercise. Experience tells me that this book will bring me much trouble, a great deal of abuse, a number of threats and considerable professional and personal inconvenience. But I firmly believe that vaccination is one of the most offensive and dangerous of all modern medical practices and I find it appalling that it is allowed to grow, seemingly unchecked and unquestioned. I don't believe anyone, anywhere, knows just how much harm is being done by the establishment's unquestioned enthusiasm for a practice which is of such doubtful value and which offers such potential for disaster. I hope this book will raise some questions and some doubts and I hope that readers will share my concerns with their families, their friends, their neighbours and their medical advisers.

*Vernon Coleman, August 2011*

# Introduction

*`The whole apparatus for spreading knowledge, the schools and the press, wireless and cinema, will be used exclusively to spread those views which, whether true or false, will strengthen the belief in the rightness of the decisions taken by the authority; and all information that might cause doubt or hesitation will be withheld.' - F. A. Hayek*

One of the most fashionable medical interventions today is undoubtedly vaccination. A generation or two ago children obtained immunity to childhood diseases (chicken pox, measles and mumps) by attending parties. If a child contracted one of the common (but relatively unthreatening) childhood diseases all the children in the neighbourhood would be invited round for tea and games. Those children attending the party who contracted the disease would put up with spots for a week or so and then recover. Parents would, probably justifiably, assume that a child who hadn't caught the disease had quite likely acquired immunity to it. The system was simple, uneventful and relatively safe and it worked because the human immune system is designed to learn from experience. When the body produces special lymphocytes to fight pathogens those lymphocytes remain sensitised to specific infections and will respond to future infections by producing antibodies. With the aid of these antibodies the body can wipe out an appropriate invading organism before the infection can take hold. When this happens the body is said to be protecting itself by having developed immunity.

These days, children have vaccinations. Loads of them. It is the fashion. It is our way. Drug companies and doctors make huge amounts of money out of it. Vaccination is all about money. Drug companies make billions. Doctors make thousands. The big question is not `Is it safe?' or `Does it work?' but `Is it profitable?'

Governments believe that by vaccinating whole populations they reduce the incidence of illness and therefore ensure that people spend more time at work and less time at home, wastefully tucked up in bed with a hot water bottle and a bottle of pills.

There are three main types of vaccine.

First, there are the live vaccines which contain an attenuated strain of a microorganism. The hope with these vaccines is that they will produce a subclinical infection. Viral vaccines may contain attenuated strains of a virus or an inactivated virus. They are prepared in tissue culture, which may contain antibiotics, or in chick embryos. These vaccines are, therefore, unsuitable for patients who are allergic to the antibiotics concerned or to egg protein. (Sadly, many doctors do not bother to ask their patients if they have any allergies which might make vaccination especially hazardous. And so these vaccines are not infrequently given inappropriately.)

Second, there are vaccines which contain killed micro-organisms. These vaccines may contain an intact (but dead) organism or a sample pack of specific antigens.

Third, bacterial toxins which have been inactivated are also used in vaccine preparation.

Vaccines can be given by mouth, nasal spray or injection but these days most are given by injection. Whatever the route or format, a vaccination is designed to give the body enough exposure to a particular pathogen to develop defence cells, but not enough of the pathogen to produce signs and symptoms of illness.

Unfortunately, this is a balancing act which the vaccine manufacturers don't always get perfectly right. And there are many potential hazards. For example, if a live vaccine is given to someone with an ineffective immune system the result can be catastrophic - and fatal.

The immunity provided by vaccines varies enormously. Some vaccines provide lifetime protection. Some vaccines fail to work and provide no protection at all.

The bottom line is that there are many things that can (and do) go wrong. Anyone who claims that all vaccines are always safe and always effective is a nincompoop - and yet that is a claim that is frequently made by British doctors and nurses.

Not surprisingly, many people are confused and worried about vaccines. They don't know what to believe. Are vaccines as safe as the Government says they are? Are they essential? Parents, in particular, can become very bewildered. Will their child die if he or she doesn't have the usual series of vaccinations? Most patients and parents are prepared to accept the Government's assurance that vaccines are safe and utterly essential; they contentedly accept what they are told. But those who want answers will probably find it difficult to get them. Many of my readers who have tried to discuss vaccines with their doctors have complained that their physicians, rude and certain in their ignorance, simply insist that vaccines are perfectly safe and that is the end of the matter.

Those GPs aren't alone in their single-minded defence of vaccination. In Britain, politicians, doctors, nurses and journalists all enthusiastically insist that vaccines are entirely safe and free from side effects. They are all either lying or ill-informed. Lest you assume that is hyperbole let me point out that when, in April 2011, the US Health Department's National Vaccine Injury Compensation Programme released its figures for 2010 the report showed that allegedly safe childhood vaccines officially killed or injured no less than 2,699 children in the year 2010 in America. The parents of those children received $110 million in damages. The US Government has reportedly also paid compensation to the parents of autistic children. And at roughly the same time the Japanese Government halted part of its own vaccination programme after a number of children had died after being vaccinated. (Can you imagine the fuss there would be if a food company marketed a product which killed or injured 2,699 healthy children in a single year? How long would they stay in business with that sort of record?)

I believe that everyone should be told the facts so that they can make up their own minds about the value of any vaccine. Deciding whether or not to have a vaccination is a big decision. It isn't something to be done lightly. The wrong decision can easily lead to a lifetime of regrets.

Sadly, one big problem is undoubtedly the fact that many doctors simply don't know very much about the safety or effectiveness of vaccines. They know what the Government tells them and they know what the company which makes the vaccine tells them. And that's it. But no sensible person trusts Governments and I don't think I am alone, or being unduly cynical, in thinking that companies making vaccines aren't a reliable source of unbiased information about the effectiveness and safety of vaccines.

`My doctor implied that I was just being stupid when I said I wasn't sure that I wanted my child vaccinated,' complained one reader of mine. `His attitude was that it had nothing to do with me and that I should just allow him to do whatever he thought best.'

`My wife came home crying,' complained another reader. `She had the temerity to question her doctor about vaccination. He told her that if she refused to have our child vaccinated he would call in the social workers since in his view our refusal to allow vaccination made us unfit to be parents. What really upset me is that my wife hadn't refused to have our child vaccinated. She just wanted to talk about it.'

This paternalistic attitude seems strong among doctors and other health workers, most of whom seem to prefer to answer any questions with abuse rather than facts. I suspect that this is a consequence of the fact that doctors and health visitors are full to the brim with ignorance and don't have any room for facts with which to answer questions. (Curiously, GPs invariably fail to mention that they have a vested financial interest in promoting vaccination.)

I believe that the whole vaccination story is one of the great modern scandals of our time. The entire medical profession (at least the part of it in general practice) has been bribed and most doctors, whether working as hospital consultants, GPs or public health officials, know very little about vaccination but simply follow the establishment line, never question what they are told by the drug industry, dismiss all critics of vaccination as dangerous lunatics and get very rich by promoting mass vaccination programmes which have never been proven to be safe or effective.

In Britain, doctors give fistfuls of potentially lethal vaccine to tiny babies with developing immune systems. They start dumping the damned stuff into babies when they are two-months-old, for heaven's sake. And yet there is no evidence proving that vaccines are safe when given in job lots like this and no evidence proving long-term safety. The absence of evidence isn't much of a surprise since no research is done to check either safety or efficacy. The establishment puts the onus on the doubters to find evidence that there are dangers, knowing that this is pretty well impossible to do without the cooperation of the drug companies, the Government or the medical establishment.

If you or I want to sell home-made sweets to kids we will have all sorts of health and safety officials crawling over us, our kitchen and our shop. But doctors merrily squirt gallons of potentially toxic junk into babies who are still breast feeding.

Where's the sense in telling nursing mothers to be aware that what they swallow will end up in their breast milk (and in their developing baby) when the Government promotes its pre-school vaccination programmes with Goebbels-like efficiency?

I fear that doctors have lost their way.

GPs receive massive payments for giving vaccinations and huge bonus payments for vaccinating large quantities of their patients. A GP who jabs enough patients gets a thumping great wodge of cash paid straight into his bank account. A GP who is questioning and discerning will be punished because he won't get the bribe money. And if he doesn't watch his back very carefully he could well find himself being nicely fried by what I believe to be the world's most entirely useless watchdog: the General Medical Council.

And so the vast majority of GPs do as they are told. Most know nothing about the dangers of the damned vaccines they so happily jab into patients' arms and I suspect that they don't want to know anything. Politicians, nurses, and journalists all bury their fears and suspicions and help bang the drum for vaccination. Question the whole damned sordid business and these ill-educated propagandists (who, like the doctors, know nothing about the risks of the toxic mixtures they are promoting) will throw up their hands in horror.

As vaccinations increase so the number of health problems caused by vaccines will soar. At the same time the link between vaccinations and illness will continue to be as strenuously denied as was the link between smoking and lung cancer.

Countries which have not yet adopted mass vaccination programmes would, perhaps, be wise to ask some serious and rather fundamental questions before starting to do so. Here are a few questions that might be asked.

Who benefits most from vaccination programmes?

Are vaccines given to protect the community or to protect the individual?

Where is the scientific evidence showing that vaccines are really effective?

Where is the long-term scientific evidence showing that vaccines are safe?

Where is the long-term scientific evidence showing that giving a ton and a half of mixed gunk into an eight-week-old baby doesn't cause brain damage?

Doctors, politicians and journalists tend to avoid answering these questions because they much prefer to perpetuate the traditional myths about vaccination and to argue that vaccines have helped us eradicate a whole host of previously deadly diseases. Moreover, they will argue that it is vaccines which we must thank for the longevity we enjoy.

All this is, to put it as politely as I feel able, utter bollocks. As I will show in this book the evidence makes it clear that diseases said to have been conquered by vaccines were in fact often controlled by other means long before vaccines were introduced. Sadly, the problem is that the doctors, politicians and drug companies who are promoting vaccination are more interested in profit than evidence.

Over the years I have learned that the truth about many aspects of medicine is suppressed and, as a result, most people simply don't know the facts. The information generally available is provided by politicians, scientists and doctors who bend the truth for commercial reasons and then repeated by journalists who simply believe, and report, what they are told. The result is that millions of people make vital decisions based on half-truths, quarter-truths and downright lies.

Anyone who insists that vaccines are safe and effective is a liar. Life is made easier for the liars because most people are overwhelmed with trying to cope with day-to-day life problems and eager to accept what appear to be comfortable certainties. They are constantly frightened and bewildered and therefore susceptible to the bleatings of reassuring tricksters. They want to trust advice from people they believe to be experts. All that makes the great betrayal even more contemptible and unforgivable.

If you try to find evidence that vaccination works you will find that the best `evidence' offered by those promoting it is that there has been a reduction in the incidence of certain diseases against which vaccination is now commonplace. This is not evidence. It is akin to claiming that there are no elephants in the centre of London because women carry handbags. It is irrelevant nonsense. The incidence of those diseases fell - and was continuing to fall - long before vaccination was introduced.

It is vaccines which, I suspect, best illustrate the recklessness and ruthlessness of the medical profession and the pharmaceutical industry and the way in which both have helped damage the human immune system.

Vaccination programmes are a particularly poignant example of the way in which doctors can do harm partly because just about every individual in the `developed' world will at some time or another be vaccinated and partly because vaccines are given to millions of perfectly healthy people. Individuals who have absolutely nothing wrong with them visit their doctor and allow themselves to be vaccinated in the belief that they are being injected with something perfectly safe which will protect them from disease in the future. Sadly, there is now a dramatic amount of evidence to show that their faith is misplaced and that vaccines may cause an enormous amount of trouble - and do serious and possibly sometimes irreparable harm to their bodies. It is hard to think of a worse global scandal.

Why do so many people assume that vaccination is a good thing? Because they are told so. And who tells them? The trio of evil. Drug companies make money out of vaccinations. And so do doctors. Politicians go along for the ride because they have been tricked and pressured into supporting vaccination by the drug companies and because it is now impossible to back out without exposing themselves (or, rather, the Government) to multi-billion pound lawsuits.

The Government bribes GPs to promote vaccination because its advisors know that more than 90 per cent coverage is required to provide herd immunity - and reduce the incidence of a disease within a community. (I will explain in this book that vaccines are given not to protect individuals against disease but to protect communities against financial loss.)

Where is the evidence that vaccination is truly safe and effective? There isn't any. On the contrary, I believe that by giving people too many vaccines we are creating massive amounts of illness. The trio of evil would do far more good by encouraging greater levels of natural immunity than they do by encouraging dependence on vaccines. Over the last 40 years I have published scores of predictions and warnings about health hazards. Most have already been proved accurate. (The only difference today is that (as I will show) my warnings and predictions are now not just ignored but also actively suppressed.) I have repeatedly criticised the official enthusiasm for vaccination.

In our new world the few doctors who do stand up and say something, and who dare to point out that vaccination programmes are a hazard and do more harm than good, are quickly silenced. They are discredited and scorned and their work is not published. I have, over the years, discovered many of the hazards of telling the truth. My books are rarely reviewed these days. Most national newspapers and magazines ban all advertisements for my books. Planned interviews are invariably cancelled before they take place. In the last ten years I have twice been mysteriously investigated at length by HMRC (on both occasions it turned out that I had paid too much tax.) And, as I show elsewhere in this book I have even been banned from speaking to groups of NHS employees. I mention all this to show just why only one-sided is the information provided for public consumption. It is hardly surprising that parents without medical training and a special interest in iatrogenesis believe the lies they are told about vaccines and think that people like me are half-baked, dangerous lunatics.

I believe that if you are giving a drug to save someone's life (and it is clear that if the drug is not tried then the patient will most certainly die) then it may be ethically acceptable to take risks. But when you are giving a vaccine to perfectly healthy individuals in order to protect the community (and the State) from inconvenience and cost then risks are not acceptable. And yet vaccines are given to millions of people without anyone really having any idea what the long-term consequences may be.

As you read through this book remember that if these facts weren't true I would either be sued or struck off the medical register. Why haven't you read the truths in this book elsewhere? Well, over the last 40 years I've made a lot of enemies who do whatever they can to ensure that the truth is suppressed. The medical establishment works hard to protect itself (and that includes the pharmaceutical industry) and to pressurise journalists into perpetuating the officially acceptable myths and lies.

As you read, remember that I have no vested interests. I don't represent anyone. If I thought vaccines were marvellous I would say so and attack the people trying to oppose their use. My only interest is the truth. My concern is that I believe that the amount of illness and the number of deaths caused by vaccinations far exceed the amount of illness and the number of deaths caused by the diseases against which vaccinations are supposed to offer protection. Remember that I have no vested interest for or against vaccines. I don't receive money from drug companies. I don't sell alternatives to vaccines. All I have to sell are my books; my only product is the truth.     The whole vaccination story is one of the great modern scandals of our time. The entire medical profession (at least the part of it in general practice) has been bribed by the Government, using taxpayers' money. In my first book *The Medicine Men* (1975) I wrote that doctors who did what the drug industry told them to do could hardly describe themselves as belonging to a profession. Even I did not then imagine just how easy it would be to bribe and buy an entire profession.

The truth is that doctors, whether working as hospital consultants, GPs or public health officials, know very little about vaccination. Most simply follow the establishment line, never question what they are told by the drug industry and dismiss all critics of vaccination as dangerous lunatics.

I've been writing about vaccines for decades and in the days when radio and television stations were allowed to interview me, and arrange debates, I often met doctors promoting the official `vaccines will save the world' line. Most of them didn't know any of the stuff in this book. They just believed what they were told by the Government and the drug industry and looked at their bank statements every month with growing pride (and perhaps a little incredulity).

Remember: everything in this book is true. Everything *they* tell you is a lie.

And ask yourself: Why has Vernon Coleman written this book? I promise you I don't need the money (if I did I could make far more money writing another book about cats). I certainly don't need the hassle. I don't *need* to write about vaccines (there are scores of other things I would find more fun to write about) and I could think of a hundred book topics that would sell better (I know from past experience that serious medical books don't usually sell very well at all). So why have I written this book? The answer is simple. I've written it because it is the truth and no one else will tell this particular truth.

I can share this truth and so I have.

# 1. The Vaccination Myth

Most practising doctors and nurses at the sharp end of medicine undoubtedly believe that vaccines have helped wipe out some of the deadliest infectious diseases. Many members of the medical profession would put vaccination high on any list of great medical discoveries. Those who promote vaccines often claim that vaccination programmes have reduced illness, prevented millions of deaths and are the main reason why the average life expectation has risen. These are all barefaced lies.

Vaccination is widely respected by doctors and others in the health care industry because of the assumption that it is through vaccination that many of the world's most lethal infectious diseases have been eradicated. But this simply isn't true: it is a myth. As I have shown in many of my books infectious diseases were conquered by the provision of cleaner drinking water and better sewage facilities. The introduction of vaccination programmes came along either just at the same time or later when the death rates from the major infectious diseases had already fallen. There really isn't any evidence to show that vaccination programmes have ever been of any real value - either to individuals or to communities.

The mythical power of vaccination programmes has for years constantly been sustained by governments and organisations announcing, apparently with complete conviction, that such and such a disease will be eradicated when the relevant vaccination programme has been completed.

The principle behind vaccination is a convincing one.

The theory is that when an individual is given a vaccine - which consists of a weakened or dead version of the disease against which protection is required - his or her body will be tricked into developing antibodies to the disease in exactly the same way that a body develops antibodies when it is exposed to the disease itself.

But in reality things aren't quite so simple. How long do the antibodies last? Do they always work? What about those individuals who don't produce antibodies at all? Vaccination, like so much of medicine, is a far more inexact science than doctors (and drug companies) would like us to think.

The truth is that it is a ruthless and self-serving lie to claim that vaccines have wiped out many diseases and have contributed hugely to the increase in life expectancy we now enjoy. The evidence shows that the diseases which are supposed to have been wiped out by vaccines were disappearing long before vaccines were introduced. And the argument that we are living longer is a statistical myth which rests upon the fact that in the past the infant mortality rate was much higher than it is now (because of contaminated drinking water and other public health problems). When the infant mortality rate is high the average life expectation is low. When the infant mortality rate falls then the average life expectation rises. (If one person dies at the age of 1 and another dies at the age of 99 they have an average life span of 50 years. If the person who died prematurely lives longer then the average life span will be much longer).

The bottom line, then, is that the evidence shows that vaccination programmes have not done the things they are credited with but have done most of the things they are blamed for. The decline in disease, the reduction in infant mortality rates and the increase in average life expectation are all due to improved living conditions. Cleaner water, efficient methods of removing sewage, fresher food, less poverty and less overcrowding are the real reasons why these improvements have taken place. Anyone who doubts this has only to look at graphs showing mortality rates and life expectation rates alongside graphs showing when vaccines were introduced. The graphs show clearly that the improvements took place before the vaccines were introduced. Study the evidence relating to whooping cough, tetanus, diphtheria, smallpox, polio and other diseases and it becomes clear that the incidence of these diseases, and number of deaths caused by them, were in decline long before the relevant vaccines were introduced.

## 2. Vaccine Bonanza

As the years have gone by the number of vaccines available has increased steadily but remorselessly.

A decade or two ago the only vaccines available were against a relatively small number of diseases including smallpox, tuberculosis, polio, cholera, diphtheria, tetanus and whooping cough. Today, the number of available vaccines seems to grow almost daily. In the past vaccines were produced against major killer diseases. Today vaccines are produced against diseases such as measles, mumps and chickenpox which have been traditionally regarded as relatively benign inconveniences of childhood.

In Britain, most children who reach their second birthday will have already received 21 vaccinations against seven different diseases. That's a hell of a lot of gunk to slosh around in a small, growing body. The routine, standard, run of the mill, no questions asked vaccination programme starts at two months (I still can't believe that). Babies just eight-weeks-old have a single jab against diphtheria, tetanus, pertussis, haemophilus influenzae type b and polio and another against pneumococcal disease. Then, as if that were not enough, babies of three months have another pile of gunk stuffed into them. And more at four months, just in case the first two batches didn't screw up their immune systems. Babies have some protection against infection from antibodies obtained from their mothers. This lasts for a few months after birth. Otherwise a baby's immune system is rather rudimentary and takes a few years to develop fully. Nevertheless, we now jab young children with a growing number of toxic vaccines. Just what do this do to the developing immune system? You will find a full list of the research papers investigating the damage done to the infant immune system by repeated vaccinations written on the palm of your left hand.

The poor little beggars then have a rest from vaccinations until they are three-years-old or so. And then they get some more. Girls of 12 or 13 have some more potent gunk stuffed into them and everyone gets another armful when they reach their teens. The rules change regularly as drug companies think of something new to flog and new vaccines are added. (Whenever the rules change it is, presumably, fair to assume that the previous vaccination regime was wrong or inadequate in some way. No one ever says this, of course.)

All this is nothing compared to the gunk sloshing around inside small Americans who will have been given more than 30 doses of 10 different vaccines before they can say 'television'. (These figures are almost certainly out of date by the time you read this. I can guarantee that the figures will be higher, not lower.) Does anyone know what happens inside the body when all these different vaccinations are given together? Do different vaccines work with or against one another? What about the risk of interactions? Exactly how does the immune system cope when it is suddenly bombarded with so much foreign material? And what about dangerous contaminants? Your guess is as good as mine and mine is as good as your doctor's. So, we're all in the dark together.

The pharmaceutical companies and doctors who profit from all this giving of vaccines are not content with the current situation. The vaccine industry never stops looking for new opportunities and researchers are constantly talking about introducing new vaccines. Although new vaccines are forever being introduced, vaccines are rarely if ever withdrawn - even though the diseases involved may be rare or mild. The drug companies can always warn: `If the vaccine isn't given then the disease will come back.'

The search for new vaccines for old diseases is endless. Some plans are imaginative. Scientists have apparently developed a banana vaccine by creating genetically engineered banana plants. There are plans to develop bananas which `protect' against hepatitis B, measles, yellow fever and poliomyelitis. Other scientists have developed a genetically engineered potato designed to be used as a vaccine against cholera. The active part of the potato remains active during the process of cooking and so a portion of genetically engineered chips could soon be a vaccine against cholera. (I am not making this up.) According to a British nursing magazine, nurses are now calling for a vaccine to help stop the norovirus. Giving a vaccine is, presumably, easier than washing your hands. Similarly, fat people are constantly demanding a vaccine to enable them to keep eating cakes without ever getting fatter. There are, so I am told, vaccines in the pipeline for just about everything ranging from asthma to earache. There is a planned genetically engineered vaccine which will provide protection against 40 different diseases. The vaccine, which will contain the raw DNA of all those different diseases, will be given to newborn babies to provide them with protection for life. Inevitably, countless scientists around the world have spent enormous amounts of money and energy trying to create a vaccine against AIDS. A vaccine that makes sex safe will be worth a fortune.

Naturally, the pharmaceutical industry is constantly searching for more and more new vaccines and wherever they spot the beginnings of a market, a demand, they will do their best to serve up something appropriate. I have lost count of the number of times I have read of researchers working on a vaccine to prevent cancer.

Meanwhile, the drug companies continue with the old faithfuls; the profitable cash cows which keep the billions pouring in. Every year new flu jabs appear on the market.

I don't know about you but I can no longer keep up with what is going on. I have long since given up trying to work out which vaccines are very dangerous and which are just a bit dangerous - and to whom. The only certainty is that manufacturing (and giving) vaccines is big business. The people who sell vaccines make a lot of money. And the doctors who give them (or who authorise nurses to give them on their behalf) make a lot of money too. Vaccination is a big, and very profitable, industry. This is vaccine bonanza time for drug companies and doctors.

## 3. What Research Is Done To Test New Vaccines?

It doesn't require a great deal of learning to realise that there must be dangers involved in injecting a potentially dangerous foreign substance directly into the body. Even an idiot can see that must be hazardous. And yet where is the evidence showing that vaccines have been tested? For example, I have not been able to find any evidence that studies have been done to prove that giving babies numerous vaccines within a short period of time is safe.

One of the problems with setting up any such research programme would undoubtedly be the problem of obtaining informed consent (an essential requirement before any new product can be tested). Obviously, an eight-week-old baby cannot give consent to being jabbed with some potentially toxic material. But how can the parents give consent for a potentially dangerous procedure, on behalf of their baby, when their baby is perfectly well? If a baby will die unless a new treatment is tried - and existing therapies have proved ineffective - then the parents are clearly justified in giving their consent. That is how new treatments are properly tested and developed. But how can parents give consent for their baby to be given a potentially dangerous vaccination when the child is perfectly healthy? And what parents would give their consent under those circumstances? When new drugs and vaccines intended for adult use are introduced they are tested on volunteers, under controlled circumstances. The guinea pigs are carefully observed. Even so there are some disasters when new pharmacological products are tested for the first time. Adult patients used as guinea pigs are well paid for the risks they take.

The bottom line is that it is, in my view, impossible for drug companies and doctors to perform ethically acceptable research to test out new vaccines designed for use on babies and children.

I suspect that if research had been done which proved that vaccines were safe then it would be published and widely promoted (if only to silence critics like myself). At the moment we must all rely on the unsupported confidence of drug companies and the doctors who give vaccinations - all of whom have a vested interest in promoting vaccination and in assuring us all that there are no risks.

Just as surprisingly, and just as shocking, is the fact that as far as I have been able to find out no long-term research has been done, or is being done, into the safety and effectiveness of vaccines. Drug companies and doctors simply assume that vaccines are safe and effective because they want them to be. I wonder how many enthusiastic supporters of vaccination know that, as far as I've been able to find out, neither doctors nor drug companies conduct long-term follow-up studies to prove that vaccines are safe. I wonder how many know that the Government doesn't bother either. It is a scandal of brobdingnagian proportions that little or no ongoing research is done to find out how safe or effective vaccines are in the long-term. Drug companies and politicians say that vaccines are safe and effective. And people believe them. Doctors (and others) who speak out against vaccines are ignored and their work is suppressed. Madness.

The basic problem is that these days research work is usually done with a specific, commercial purpose in mind. Research into new products is begun under the guidance and approval of drug companies and the aim is to obtain some useful results which can be used to promote a particular product. What drug company is going to pay for research which might show that its product kills people? Most doctors who do research have links to drug companies and aren't likely to bite the hands that feed them so well. Even if a research programme did show that a vaccine was unsafe the results would be unlikely to be published. Drug companies have a track record of suppressing inconvenient or commercially damaging research results. And, of course, it is very easy to `fiddle' research in order to prove a particular point. By redefining diseases, by choosing patients selectively, by diagnosing diseases in a different way and so on it is possible to `prove' whatever you want to prove.

Without impartial Government support it is extremely unlikely that anyone will conduct research designed to find out whether or not vaccines are safe and effective. And the Government is not going to pay for any research designed to find out just how safe and effective vaccines really are because the Government also has a vested interest in maintaining the myth that vaccines are safe and effective.

The result is that many of the scientific papers which do discuss vaccination have been written by scientists working for the Government (which promotes vaccination) or the drug companies (which make the stuff). These links are not always made clear when the papers are published - and even if the links are revealed does that really make a difference? Many of the people who do research on vaccines, and who sit on committees deciding which vaccines should be given and when, have strong financial connections with drug companies but we are expected to accept that their links with the drug companies in no way affect their judgements or decisions about the use of vaccines. The researchers publishing most of the work on vaccines are unlikely to risk being contaminated by cooperating with independent thinkers; most are employed by, or in some other way linked to, the Government or the drug industry.

There is a mass of evidence showing that vaccines are potentially dangerous. There is no shortage of evidence showing that vaccines make a good many healthy people ill. And there is a frightening amount of evidence supporting the claim that vaccines kill people. It is even fairly easy to prove that vaccines have had no significant effect on the incidence of many of the diseases they are supposed to prevent.

But I haven't been able to find evidence proving that vaccines are effective. Doctors happily jab stuff into the arms of the perfectly healthy without evidence proving that what they are doing will save lives.

It is simply not good enough for doctors to just say that vaccines are safe and effective because they want them to be. When you are injecting the stuff into millions of kids there ought to be tons of research which proves this conclusively.

Incidentally, if you would like to assess the quality of the information proving that vaccines are safe and effective you can easily do this for yourself. Simply use your favourite search engine to investigate these two questions: `What scientific research has been done to prove that vaccines are really safe?' and `What scientific research has been done to prove that vaccines are effective?'. (Phrase your questions in any way you like, of course. I don't want you to feel that I'm leading you in any particular direction. And check the source of whatever you find.)

Finally, here's a simple, cheap to perform, clinical trial that would tell us whether or not individual vaccines are safe and effective.

All doctors have to do is to make a note of how many children who receive a vaccine develop that disease and then compare those results with the number of children who get the disease but haven't had the vaccine. This will provide information showing that the vaccine is (or is not) effective.

And they could make a note of the number of vaccinated children who develop serious health problems after vaccination and then compare that number with the incidence of serious health problems among unvaccinated children. What could be easier than that?

These would be easy and cheap trials to perform. They would simply require the collection of some basic information. And it would be vital to follow the children for at least 20 years to obtain useful information. A trial involving 100,000 children would be enough.

But I do not know of anyone who has done, or is doing, this simple research. Could it possibly be that no one does such basic research because the results might be embarrassing for those who want to sell vaccines?

## 4. Can We Learn From Research Using Animals?

Many, if not all, of the vaccines in popular use today have at some stage in their development been tested on animals. Crucial work designed to show whether a new product is safe for human use is often performed on animals. And yet, the evidence shows that the use of animals for research is particularly nonsensical and dangerous (as well as being unutterably cruel).

Drug companies and researchers like using animals because they cannot lose. If, when a drug is being tested on animals, it appears that the animal is harmed then the drug company will say: `This is of no consequence, since animals are different to humans'. They will then sell the drug for use on people. My book *Betrayal of Trust* contains a list of several dozen drugs which cause cancer and other serious disorders in animals but which are sold for human use. When a drug is tested on animals and there are no side effects the drug company concerned will say that this proves that the drug is safe for people. This system means that they cannot lose! What is the point in testing drugs on animals? Only the drug companies gain. It is far better to test new drugs on human tissues in the laboratory than it is to test drugs for people on mice. Such tests are easier, quicker, cheaper and far more reliable than animal tests. The problem is that drug companies don't like such tests because they mean that many potentially dangerous drugs are thrown out by the testing and can never be sold.

The evidence clearly shows that animal experiments are a complete waste of time, that animal experiments have never led to any useful breakthroughs and that they are never likely to lead to any useful breakthroughs. Despite this, much of the research work done on vaccines is performed on animals.

A standard test used on rats gives results which can be accurately applied to human beings just 38 per cent of the time. This means that 62 per cent of the time the results obtained through animal experiments are wrong. Since tossing a coin would give a long-term 50 per cent chance of accuracy it would clearly be quicker, more effective, more efficient and cheaper for these scientists to spend their working days sitting around tossing coins to assess the safety of chemicals. (`Yes! Heads! We can give this to patients! No! Tails! Patients can't take that one.') But, in political and financial terms, tossing a coin would certainly not be as useful as using animals. Consider tobacco, for example. The link between tobacco and cancer was identified many years ago by doctors whose observations and research work had involved human patients. But long after doctors had established the link between tobacco and cancer in humans, animal researchers were still forcing dogs to smoke, and painting tobacco tar on the backs of mice, in attempts to show whether or not there was a laboratory link between tobacco and cancer. Politicians who wanted to avoid taking action against the wealthy and big tax paying tobacco companies were able to do so on the grounds that they were still awaiting laboratory confirmation of the link between tobacco and cancer. Decades of vague, inconclusive and contradictory results enabled the world's tobacco industry to keep selling a product which was responsible for approximately one third of all cancer deaths and which, over the years, must have been responsible for more deaths, disease and misery than any other product ever invented.

Vivisectors provide a perfect example of what psychologists call 'confirmatory bias'. They collect together all the evidence that supports their thesis and then ignore the evidence that is left - the stuff that doesn't support their belief. If pushed into a corner they delight in confusing the issue in every way they can.

To summarise: my argument against vivisection is very simple and there is no answer to it. I actually have two main arguments. First, drugs are allowed onto the market even if they cause problems in animals - on the grounds that animals are different to humans. And drugs which don't cause problems in the tested animals are allowed onto the market on the grounds that they have been proved safe. Second, the vivisectors admit that over half of their experiments on animals are unreliable and worthless. But they also admit that they don't know which of their experiments are in the minority which, they claim, may be useful. So, they clearly don't ever know which of their experiments may be of value. And if you don't know which experiments are of value then all of them are useless.

Those are the arguments I used when giving evidence at the House of Commons and the House of Lords. No one said anything in opposition to these arguments. Not a word. (That's why vivisectors now refuse to debate with me.) Moreover, when the House of Lords committee sent me the evidence offered by the Department of Health in support of vivisection I was able to destroy, systematically and logically, every shred of their evidence. I proved all their arguments in favour of vivisection to be entirely fallacious and nonsensical. I proved, without any shadow of doubt, that vivisection is worse than useless - it is dangerous. (My demolition of the Government's evidence `supporting' vivisection appears on my website www.vernoncoleman.com)

I confess that I was not terribly impressed by the peers who sat on the House of Lords committee on animals. It was a not unpleasant experience. As a witness I was treated with courtesy. It was like being on trial without the inconvenience of being sent to prison if things go badly. One of the peers was someone called Mary Warnock who wrote a book entitled *Nature and Mortality*. This is what she wrote about the committee in her book: `The reason that this committee is such fun is that it is possible, indeed necessary, to discuss these fundamental issues...Our trip to the United States was enormously enjoyable, and I look back on it as a time of endless laughter.' She described the clerk to the committee as very young and having read music at Cambridge. `We quite often meet,' she wrote, `and discuss the business, usually ending in laughter.' She concluded: 'One way and another, it will be a sad day when `Animals' disappears as an entry in my diary.' She clearly had doubts about the value of the committee: `Whether what we recommend will make any difference to the practices of the Home Office is more than doubtful,' she wrote.

She was right to be doubtful.

The truth is that the Home Office seems to me to be quite uninterested in facts or scientific evidence. The politicians and officials there (though paid by taxpayers) appear to strive only to keep the drug companies happy. Indeed, the whole establishment seems determined to do everything it can to squash opposition to vivisection. The establishment was helped in this aim when the whole anti-vivisection movement was demonised in the 1980s and 1990s by Special Branch and MI5 who had no enemy to justify their massive budgets and had to invent one. They chose anti-vivisectionists even though they must have known damned well that there was never any real danger from them. The whole a/v movement was (and is) disorganised and consisted largely of little old ladies and teenagers handing out badly printed leaflets on street corners on Saturdays. Nevertheless, the Government gave the whole lunacy official backing and a Home Secretary (Jack Straw) described animal rights activists as terrorists. I suspect that the security forces claimed that animal rights activists were a major threat to the nation simply to justify their expensive, ungoverned existence. And so, honest old ladies in brogues and tweeds and well-intentioned teenage vegans in cardboard shoes and thin waterproof jackets became the world's most unlikely and least threatening terrorists.

It is worthwhile pointing out that there is growing evidence to support the contention that many of today's new and most threatening viral epidemics have been generated by medical scientists working with animals. During the 1960's and 1970's, cancer researchers and scientists working for the military on the development of death bugs were developing HIV-like viruses in laboratories.

Misled by animal studies which suggested that viruses were responsible for the development of cancer, researchers were trying to find an anti-cancer vaccine. They combined viruses which were known to cause cancer in animals in an attempt to create new viruses which they hoped would give them some clues about how viruses caused cancer.

At the same time researchers working for the military were using animals in their attempts to develop viral weapons with which opponents could be killed (and their countries destabilised) en masse.

Because of incompetence (a common fault among the mass of second rate scientists around the world who routinely perform experiments on animals) the new viruses have been inadvertently spread through our communities.

And, of course, there is convincing evidence to suggest that AIDS was created in an animal research laboratory.

The conclusion of any independent observer has to be that vivisectors are, as a group, ignorant, unthinking, entirely selfish varlets who do as much harm to people as they do to animals. They refuse to discuss or debate what they do but rely on misinformation and propaganda. And there is a real risk that the work done by vivisectors is extremely dangerous to human health.

It is worth remembering that the biggest survey of doctors ever conducted showed that the majority of practising doctors agree that animal experiments are of no value whatsoever to patients and that patients would suffer fewer side effects if new drugs were tested on human cell and tissue cultures. Naturally, neither the medical establishment nor the media have shown much interest in these inconvenient views. A few years ago I was President of an organisation of over 1,000 doctors who opposed vivisection. The only time I was interviewed by the British media I was subjected to what I can only describe as a lengthy and subjective sneer from a presenter called Melvyn Bragg on a BBC radio programme called *Start the Week*. Bragg seemed to me to be more enthusiastic about pouring scorn on the anti-vivisection argument rather than actually listening to it.

Cruel experiments on animals in laboratories have certainly helped the drug industry and the medical profession make a great deal of money (and, do a great deal of damage to millions of unsuspecting human patients) but they haven't been of value to doctors genuinely interested in preventing (or treating) disease.

But, ironically, animals have helped us refine our views about vaccination in a rather unsuspected way. The argument that vaccines do more harm than good is strongly supported by our experiences with animals. For example, between 1968 and 1988 there were considerably more outbreaks of foot and mouth disease in countries where vaccination against foot and mouth disease was compulsory than in countries where there were no such regulations. Epidemics of foot and mouth disease always started in countries where vaccination was compulsory. If this experience with animals can be extrapolated to humans then it clearly shows that the alleged advantage to the community of vaccinating individuals simply does not exist.

Similar observations were made about the hyena dog, which was in 1989 threatened with extinction. Scientists vaccinated individual animals to protect them against rabies but more than a dozen packs then died within a year - of rabies. This happened even in areas where rabies had never been seen before. When researchers tried using a non-infectious form of the pathogen (to prevent the deaths of the remaining animals) all members of seven packs of dogs disappeared. It seems curious that the rabies vaccine is now compulsory in many parts of the world. Could it be possible that it is the vaccine which is keeping this disease alive?

# 5. Vaccination Against Diphtheria

Vaccination against diphtheria was introduced to Germany in 1925. After the introduction of the vaccine, the number of cases of diphtheria steadily increased until, shortly after the Second World War, production of the vaccine was halted. There was a decline in the incidence of the disease which coincided with the fact that the vaccination was no longer being used. When the vaccine was subsequently reintroduced the decline in the incidence of the disease slowed down.

As with whooping cough, tetanus and other diseases the incidence, and number of deaths from diphtheria, had been in decline long before the vaccine was introduced.

# 6. Vaccination Against Influenza

On January 13th 2011, newspapers carried headlines telling readers that the death toll from flu had more than doubled and had risen to 112. There were calls for compulsory vaccination against swine flu. In fact, these figures show that less people than usual were dying from flu for the time of the year. On the following day doctors and journalists described the incidence of flu as `a pandemic' and called for all children to be vaccinated immediately (despite the fact that it was mainly elderly people who were dying). Scaremongering, vaccine-promoting supporters of the planned vaccination programme pointed out that the vaccine cost only £6 per person.

Up until a year or two ago the World Health Organisation used to describe a pandemic as a disease which (among other things) killed large numbers of people.

This definition was changed in 2009 so that a disease which spread across national borders (but didn't necessarily kill many people) could be described as a pandemic.

Shortly after the definition was changed, swine flu was officially declared a serious level 6 pandemic. And countries all over the world had little choice but to start buying up huge stocks of H1N1 flu vaccine. The financial cost was enormous. And the profits for the drug companies flogging the vaccines were enormous too.

When the swine flu vaccine was first introduced it was said that it would prevent the disease. Then it was announced that it would shorten the duration of the disease. It was said that 159 deaths had occurred in Mexico as a result of the flu but this was later corrected to just seven deaths. Independent doctors warned that for children the side effects of the drug far outweighed the benefits and that one in twenty children was suffering from nausea or vomiting (severe enough to bring on dehydration) and also nightmares. The disease was being diagnosed on the NHS telephone line (provided as an alternative to a disappearing GP service) by telephone operators who were, presumably, satisfied that their diagnostic skills enabled them to differentiate between flu and early signs of other, more deadly disorders such as meningitis. (Making diagnoses on the telephone is a dangerous business even for a doctor.)

Senior politicians in Europe subsequently called H1N1 a faked pandemic and accused pharmaceutical companies (and their lackeys) of encouraging a false scare. Limited health resources had been wasted buying millions of doses of vaccine. And millions of healthy people had been needlessly exposed to the unknown side effects of vaccines that in my view had been insufficiently tested.

As always, vaccinations were given with greatest enthusiasm to children and the elderly - the most immunologically vulnerable and the easiest to damage with vaccines.

We don't develop immunity to influenza and the common cold because the viruses that cause these diseases are constantly mutating and changing. And for the same reason the anti-flu vaccine will be useless within months, weeks or days. For the drug companies this is great news because it means they can insist that everyone who is vaccinated needs revaccinating regularly.

The strains of influenza virus used are the available strains which the drug companies and the authorities guess might be the ones which will hit in the current year. The chances are, of course, that the strains of flu which will spread will be quite different.

Because the flu virus is constantly changing, scientists have to try to predict which strains are likely to produce an epidemic a year ahead. This a bit like forecasting the weather a year ahead. Actually, it's not a bit like that. It's exactly like that.

Moreover, for the sake of economic convenience, drug companies, politicians and doctors often talk about `this year's flu vaccine' as though the flu virus mutates just once a year. This, of course, is nonsense. Viruses don't take any notice of the calendar. They change as much as they like and as often as they can. The idea of giving anti-flu jabs on an annual basis is arbitrary and entirely unscientific. Once the drug companies have got hooked on an annual financial bonanza they will suggest that vaccines be given biannually. And doctors, who also make huge sums out of giving flu vaccinations, will be equally enthusiastic.

The vaccination programme is all about money.

I wonder how many people who have the flu jab know just what they are allowing their doctor (or, more likely, a nurse) to dump in their arm? How many know that a pretty standard influenza vaccine may contain: different strains of influenza viruses propagated in chicken embryos; formaldehyde (used as a preservative); polyethylene glycol (used to stimulate the immune system); gelatin (made from cows' bones) and thimerosal (which contains mercury).

In 2011, studies suggested that innate immunity is vital to flu resistance and that alveolar macrophages help to clear the flu virus out from the lungs. University of Texas researchers announced that enhancing this natural action would increase the body's resistance to flu infection. The obvious thing to do, therefore, is to encourage people to improve their natural immunity by avoiding activities which are bad for the immune system and by eating foods which help the immune system. In contrast, the whole principle of vaccination is to encourage fake immunity. But does multiple vaccination increase or lower the body's general immunity? Personally, I believe vaccination could well lower real immunity. I don't think I'm the only doctor who worries about this. When I was in practice as a GP I don't think I ever met a doctor who had an anti-flu vaccination himself (or gave one to members of his family). To be honest, I would be most unwilling to trust the judgement of such a doctor if I ever found one.

The big question which no one answers (and hardly anyone asks) is: could the widespread use of flu vaccine be spreading flu, encouraging the developing of more potent viruses and, therefore, be responsible for the fact that a surprising number of relatively young, and healthy, individuals are now dying from the disease? I don't know. And I don't believe anyone else does, either. What I do know is that flu jabs don't have any useful effect on preventing hospitalisation, death or time off work.

## 7. Vaccination Against Poliomyelitis

Doctors trying to promote vaccines often claim that the disease poliomyelitis was eradicated by the use of a vaccine. This is, to put it politely, a barefaced lie. I know facts are unfashionable with the medical establishment these days but the hard evidence shows quite conclusively that the polio vaccine has endangered vast numbers of healthy people, still kills healthy people and played no part in eradicating the disease.

Proof that the introduction of the polio vaccine wasn't the success it is often made out to be isn't difficult to find. In Tennessee, USA, the number of polio victims the year before vaccination became compulsory was 119. The year after vaccination was introduced the figure rose to 386. In North Carolina, the number of cases before vaccination was introduced was 78, while the number after the vaccine became compulsory rose to 313. There are similar figures for other American states. If you don't believe me, check out the figures. The evidence isn't that hard to find. In America, as a whole, the incidence of polio increased dramatically (by around 50 per cent) after the introduction of mass immunisation. The number of deaths from polio had fallen dramatically before the first polio vaccine was introduced.

The truth is that as with other infectious diseases the significance of polio dropped as better sanitation, better housing, cleaner water and more food were all made available in the second half of the 19th century. It was social developments rather than medical ones which increased human resistance to infectious diseases.

But the profitable vaccine is still popular. Today, paralysis caused by poliomyelitis is unheard of in many countries. But every year there are cases of paralysis probably caused by the oral polio vaccine.

However, whether or not the polio vaccine actually works is, for many people, a relatively unimportant health issue.

Of far more significance is the fact (revealed in my book *Why Animal Experiments Must Stop* in 1991) that millions of people who were given polio jabs as children in the 1950s and 1960s may now be at a greatly increased risk of developing cancer.

The problem is that although the first breakthrough in the development of a poliomyelitis vaccine was made in 1949 with the aid of a human tissue culture, when the first practical vaccine was prepared in the 1950's monkey kidney tissue was used because that was standard laboratory practice. Researchers didn't realise that one of the viruses commonly found in monkey kidney cells can cause cancer in humans.

If human cells had been used to prepare the vaccine (as they could and should have been and as they are now) the original poliomyelitis vaccine would have been much safer.

(As a side issue this is yet another example of the stupidity of using animal tissue in the treatment of human patients. The popularity of using transplants derived from animals suggests that doctors and scientists have learned nothing from this error. I sometimes despair of those who claim to be in the healing profession. Most members of the medical establishment don't have the brains required for a career in street cleaning.)

Bone, brain, liver and lung cancers have all been linked to the monkey kidney virus SV40 and something like 17 million people who were given the polio vaccine in the 1950s and 1960s are probably now at risk (me included). Moreover, there now seems to be evidence that the virus may be passed on to the children of those who were given the contaminated vaccine. The SV40 virus from the polio vaccine has already been found in cancers which have developed both in individuals who were given the vaccine as protection against polio and in the children of individuals who were given the vaccine. It seems inconceivable that the virus could have got into the tumours other than through the polio vaccine.

The American Government was warned of this danger back in 1956 but the doctor who made the discovery was ignored and her laboratory was closed down. Surprise, surprise. It was five years after this discovery before drug companies started screening out the virus. And even then Britain had millions of doses of the infected polio vaccine in stock. There is no evidence that the Government withdrew the vaccine and so it was almost certainly just used until it had all gone. No one can be sure about this because in Britain the official records which would have identified those who had received the contaminated vaccine were all destroyed by the Department of Health in 1987. Oddly enough the destruction of those documents means that no one who develops cancer as a result of a vaccine they were given (and which was recommended to their parents by the Government) can take legal action against the Government. Gosh. The world is so full of surprises. My only remaining question is a simple one: How do these bastards sleep at night?

Oh, I do have one other question.

Did your doctor, practice nurse or eager health visitor mention any of this when extolling the virtues of vaccination?

## 8. Vaccination Against Smallpox

One of the medical profession's greatest boasts is that it eradicated smallpox through the use of the smallpox vaccine. I myself believed this claim for many years. But it simply isn't true.

One of the worst smallpox epidemics of all time took place in England between 1870 and 1872 - nearly two decades after compulsory vaccination was introduced. After this evidence that smallpox vaccination didn't work the people of Leicester in the English Midlands refused to have the vaccine any more. When the next smallpox epidemic struck in the early 1890s the people of Leicester relied upon good sanitation and a system of quarantine. There was only one death from smallpox in Leicester during that epidemic. In contrast the citizens of other towns (who had been vaccinated) died in vast numbers.

Obligatory vaccination against smallpox was introduced in Germany as a result of state by-laws, but these vaccination programmes had no influence on the incidence of the disease. On the contrary, the smallpox epidemic continued to grow and in 1870 Germany had the gravest smallpox epidemic in its history. At that point the new German Reich introduced a new national law making vaccination against smallpox an even stricter legal requirement. The police were given the power to enforce the new law.

German doctors (and medical students) are taught that it was the Reich Vaccination Law which led to a dramatic reduction in the incidence of smallpox in Germany. But a close look at the figures shows that the incidence of smallpox had already started to fall before the law came into action. And the legally enforced national smallpox vaccination programme did not eradicate the disease.

Doctors and drug companies may not like it but the truth is that surveillance, quarantine and better living conditions got rid of smallpox - not the smallpox vaccine.

When the international campaign to rid the world of smallpox was at its height the number of cases of smallpox went up each time there was a large scale (and expensive) mass vaccination of populations in susceptible countries. As a result of this the strategy was changed. Mass vaccination programmes were abandoned and replaced with surveillance, isolation and quarantine.

The myth that smallpox was eradicated through a mass vaccination programme is just that - a myth. Smallpox was eradicated through identifying and isolating patients with the disease.

Jenner's work *may* have helped end smallpox's reign of terror (though better living conditions played a far more important part), but vaccination has been subsequently wildly over-promoted and over-used to prevent far less threatening disorders. Vaccinators have extrapolated from Jenner's work and built a multistorey building on nothing more substantial than a clumsily thrown together dung heap. Those whose enthusiasm for vaccination remains undimmed should perhaps be aware that Jenner himself had his own reservations. He tried out the first smallpox vaccination on his own 10-month-old son. Tragically, his son remained mentally retarded until his death at the age of 21. Jenner, the revered hero of pro-vaccination freaks, refused to have his second child vaccinated. Curiously, the doctors who talk so knowledgeably about Jenner's work on vaccination never seem to know any of this stuff.

The profession which had originally rejected Jenner's discovery as too dangerous, embraced it with diminishing reservations and unbridled enthusiasms, ignoring the risks and side effects as the profits to be made (both by the manufacturing industry and the medical profession) grew and grew; the glimpse of unending profits encouraging the development of too many vaccines which were neither effective nor safe.

As a postscript I should mention that when Louis XV contracted smallpox he is said to have survived only because his nurse hid him from the doctors who had killed his father and brother with their `treatments'. Wise nurse.

# 9. Vaccination Against Tuberculosis

Vaccination against tuberculosis is often given as the reason why this disease stopped being quite the threat to life that it had been.

But this isn't true.

Robert Koch discovered the pathogen that causes TB back in 1883. After that BCG vaccination was introduced and then, subsequently, mass treatment programmes were devised with chemotherapy. None of these discoveries or introductions had a significant effect on the incidence of tuberculosis.

Contracting TB doesn't provide any immunity against a second infection. And if a natural infection doesn't provide protection then a vaccination certainly won't provide protection. How on earth can it?

It was noticed decades ago that in the lung sanatoriums that specialised in the treatment of TB patients there was no difference in the survival rates of patients who had been `protected' against TB with BCG vaccination when compared to the survival rates of patients who had received no such `protection'.

The tuberculosis vaccination (the Bacillus Calmette-Guerin - known as BCG) consists of a weakened, living bovine mycobacteria. The vaccine was used for many years but a trial in India showed that the vaccine offers no protection against the disease. Indeed, when new cases of tuberculosis increased annually in the area where people had been vaccinated against the disease the trial seemed to suggest that there might be a link between the vaccine and outbreaks of the disease.

Many countries have now abandoned the TB vaccine - and have no plans to reintroduce it even though the disease is now once again a major health problem.

# 10. Vaccination Against Whooping Cough (aka Pertussis)

Throughout the 1970s and the 1980s I was a passionate critic of a number of vaccines - most notably the whooping cough vaccine.

The story of the whooping cough vaccine provides us with a remarkable example of dishonesty and deceit in medicine.

There has been controversy about the whooping cough vaccine for many years but in the UK the Department of Health and Social Security has consistently managed to convince the majority of medical and nursing staff to support the official line that the vaccine is both safe and effective. The official line has for years paid little attention to the facts. Put bluntly, successive governments have consistently lied about the risks and problems associated with the whooping cough vaccine.

I will explain exactly *why* I think that governments have lied to their employers (the public) a little later. For the time being I would like to concentrate on the history.

The first point that should be made is that although official spokesmen claim otherwise, I don't believe the whooping cough vaccine has ever had a significant influence on the number of children dying from whooping cough. The dramatic fall in the number of deaths caused by the disease came well before the vaccine was widely available and was, historians agree, the result of improved public health measures and the use of antibiotics.

It was in 1957 that the whooping cough vaccine was first introduced nationally in Britain - although the vaccine was tried out in the late 1940s and the early 1950s. But the incidence of whooping cough, and the number of children dying from the disease, had both fallen very considerably well before 1957. So, for example, while doctors reported 170,000 cases of whooping cough in 1950 they reported only about 80,000 cases in 1955. The introduction of the vaccine really didn't make very much, if any, difference to the fall in the incidence of the disease. Thirty years after the introduction of the vaccine, whooping cough cases were still running at about 1,000 a week in Britain.

Similarly, the figures show that the introduction of the vaccine had no effect on the number of children dying from whooping cough. The mortality rate associated with the disease had been falling appreciably since the early part of the 20th century and rapidly since the 1930s and 1940s - showing a particularly steep decline after the introduction of the sulphonamide drugs. Whooping cough is undoubtedly an extremely unpleasant disease but it has not been a major killer for many years. Successive governments have frequently forecast fresh whooping cough epidemics but none of the forecast epidemics has produced the devastation predicted.

My second point is that the whooping cough vaccine is neither very efficient nor is it safe. The efficiency of the vaccine is of subsidiary interest - although thousands of children who have been vaccinated do still get the disease - for the greatest controversy surrounds the safety of the vaccine. The DHSS has always claimed that serious adverse reactions to the whooping cough vaccine are extremely rare and the official suggestion has been that the risk of a child being brain damaged by the vaccine is no higher than one in 100,000. Leaving aside the fact that I find a risk of one in 100,000 unacceptable, it is interesting to examine this figure a little more closely, for after a little research work it becomes clear that the figure of one in 100,000 is a guess.

Numerous researchers have studied the risks of brain damage following whooping cough vaccination and their results make fascinating reading. Between 1960 and 1981, for example, nine reports were published showing that the risk of brain damage varied between one in 6,000 and one in 100,000. The average was a risk of one in 50,000. It is clear from these figures that the Government simply chose the figure which showed the whooping cough vaccine to be least risky. Moreover, the one in 100,000 figure was itself an estimate - a guess.

Although the British Government consistently claims that whooping cough is a dangerous disease, the figures show that it is not the indiscriminate killer it is made out to be. Whooping cough causes very few deaths a year in Britain. Many more deaths are caused by tuberculosis and meningitis.

The truth about the whooping cough vaccine is that it has, in the past, been a disaster.

The vaccine has been withdrawn in some countries because of the amount of brain damage associated with its use. In Japan, Sweden and West Germany the vaccine has, in the past, been omitted from regular vaccination schedules. In America, some years ago, two out of three whooping cough vaccine manufacturers stopped making the vaccine because of the cost of lawsuits. On 6th December 1985 the *Journal of the American Medical Association* published a major report showing that the whooping cough vaccine was, without doubt, linked to the development of serious brain damage.

The final nail in the coffin lid is the fact that the British Government quietly paid out compensation to the parents of hundreds of children who had been brain damaged by the whooping cough vaccine. Some parents who accepted damages in the early years were given £10,000. Later the sum was raised to £20,000.

My startling conclusion is that for many years now the whooping cough vaccine has been killing or severely injuring more children than the disease itself. In the decade after 1979, around 800 children (or their parents) received money from the Government as compensation for vaccine produced brain damage. In the same period less than 100 children were killed by whooping cough. I think that made the vaccine more dangerous than the disease. And that, surely is quite unacceptable. So, *why* did the British Government continue to encourage doctors to use the vaccine?

There are two possible explanations. The first explanation is the more generous of the two and concerns the Government's responsibility for the health of the community as a whole. The theory here is that by encouraging millions of parents to have their children vaccinated the Government can reduce the incidence of the disease in the community. In the long run this (theoretically) reduces the risk of there being any future epidemics of whooping cough. In other words the Government risks the lives of individual children for the good of the next generation.

The second, less charitable explanation is that the British Government was looking after its own interests by continuing to claim that the whooping cough vaccine was safe enough to use. If the British Government had withdrawn the whooping cough vaccine, it would have been admitting that the vaccine was dangerous. And it would obviously have had to pay out a great deal of money in compensation. By a good deal I mean billions. Lots of billions.

Whatever explanation you consider most accurate, the unavoidable fact is that the Government has, in the past, consistently lied about the whooping cough vaccine, has distorted the truth and has deceived both the medical profession (for the majority of doctors and nurses who give these injections accept the recommendations made by the Government without question) and millions of parents.

The British Government may have saved itself a tidy sum in damages. But the cost to the nation's health has been enormous.

And today no one with anything resembling a functioning brain believes anything the Government says about vaccines or, indeed, anything else.

The whooping cough vaccine used to be given to older children but young babies (who had not been vaccinated) still died from the disease (although the so-called experts claimed that by giving the vaccine to older children the disease would be eradicated and babies would not get it). So now they give the vaccine to eight-week-old babies and hope not too many of them die and that when babies do die no one can prove it's the vaccine.

How many children will be killed by the vaccine? Will Arsenal win the 2020 FA Cup? Will Tony Blair ever be imprisoned for war crimes? These are all imponderables. For the answers, we must wait.

## 11. Vaccines Are Designed To Protect the Community

Governments are enthusiastic about vaccination not because the politicians want to protect citizens from illness (when have Governments ever cared a jot about individuals?) but because they believe that vaccinations help prevent the spread of disease within a community. They're wrong, but that's what they've been told and that's what they believe.

The idea is a simple one.

The theory is that if enough children (or, indeed, adults) are vaccinated then the incidence of a disease is likely to be lower. Vaccinations don't by any means provide complete protection (many children who are vaccinated still develop the diseases against which they have been vaccinated) but the hope is that they may cut down the incidence of a disease.

And the advantage to a Government is obvious. If, instead of a million children being ill with measles just half a million develop the disease then the number of parents having time off work will be reduced accordingly. Vaccination programmes are favoured by Governments because they ease the economic burden on the State. Vaccinations are given not to prevent death or serious injury (the diseases against which most vaccines are now given do not usually kill or seriously injure) but to protect the community.

Here's the deal: Child A is vaccinated to stop children B and C getting the disease and to stop the parents of B and C needing to take time off work. So it is, as usual with vaccination, all about money. The aim is to help maximise the State's income. But it is, of course, Child A who takes all the risk.

If you're a public-spirited parent then you perhaps won't mind risking your child's health for the sake of the State.

But it would be nice if they told you all this, wouldn't it?

Maybe they don't because, deep, deep down, they rather suspect that most parents would be touched by unpatriotic reluctance when expected to risk their child's health for the sake of the nation (or, more accurately, our EU region).

The philosophy behind vaccination programmes is remarkably ruthless. The State comes first. The individual comes nowhere.

Let me explain it another way: if you could cure all present cancers and prevent anyone ever getting cancer again by performing an experiment on one healthy child, would you go ahead - knowing that the child would certainly die? Would you sacrifice an innocent and perfectly healthy child for the good of the community?

Let's make it more interesting.

Let's assume that the child is yours.

The dilemma is now a simple one.

If you allow scientists to kill your child then no one will ever again develop cancer.

Would you allow them to kill your child?

Well, that's the decision the Government has already made on your behalf by electing to recommend (or insist) that your child be vaccinated. They are pushing vaccination not for your child's benefit but for the good of the community. But they didn't bother to ask you what you thought about it. Instead they lied to you - telling you that the vaccinations were for your child's benefit.

Not many people realise that vaccination programmes are primarily designed to reduce the incidence of infection in the community, rather than keeping individual children healthy. I wonder how many of those who promote vaccination so enthusiastically realise that children are put at risk to protect the community. Politicians don't tell parents the truth about this because they suspect (probably rightly) that many parents would refuse to have their children vaccinated if they knew. The bottom line is that Governments promote vaccination for financial reasons. They believe that if they persuade citizens to be vaccinated (and to have their children vaccinated) then the incidence of infectious disease will be lower and workers will need less time off work.

Knowing all this, do politicians have their children vaccinated? Well, that's where it gets interesting because politicians who use their children at every possible opportunity suddenly become shy and reticent when asked if their children have been vaccinated. `You can't possibly ask me that,' they say indignantly. `My children are private individuals.' And then two weeks later they talk endlessly about their children's illnesses in order to deflect criticism of some outrageous piece of behaviour, or they pose with their children in order to help win a vote or two or to deflect criticism of some indefensible Government policy. Most senior politicians are just bright enough not to have their children vaccinated, and even when vaccinations become compulsory (as they will) they will find a way to avoid them. Politicians are ruthless. They will kill your children in the hope of cutting community costs (and in the certainty of pleasing drug companies). But, for some reason, they are less enthusiastic about killing their own. And do doctors have their children vaccinated? Well, most aren't saying and that, in itself, is pretty telling.

Nothing is going to force politicians to change their view. First, the cost of looking after individuals who have been brain damaged by vaccination usually falls onto families, rather than the Government. It is parents who, more often than not, take on the huge financial, physical and emotional burden of caring for a vaccine damaged child. And second, Governments have promoted vaccines and vaccination programmes with such fervour that they cannot now back pedal. If they did they would expose themselves to vast, multi-billion pound lawsuits. Governments are now firmly committed to vaccination and politicians aren't going to change their views about vaccines. Politicians, doctors and drug companies are joined together irreversibly.

# 12. Compulsory Vaccination

Enthusiasm for vaccination has become almost hysterical in much of the world. Drug companies promote vaccination programmes because they make billions out of vaccines. Doctors are equally enthusiastic because they can charge huge fees for vaccinating their patients. And Governments everywhere are enthusiastic because they have been told (by drug companies and doctors) that vaccination programmes help prevent disease and therefore save money.

But vaccination is, in my considered view, a massive confidence trick.

And there is now much talk in America and Europe of compulsory vaccination programmes being introduced.

Compulsory vaccinations have already been introduced in some areas of the world and in Britain some general practitioners (GPs) are already refusing to look after patients if they don't agree to have their children vaccinated. There is a simple, selfish financial reason for this. If patients refuse vaccination, British family doctors lose out on huge cash bonuses.

I now have no doubt that despite the dangers and inefficiencies known to be associated with it, vaccination will become compulsory in the West. The hazards and inadequacies will be ignored. It will not be the first time. Compulsory vaccination was introduced in Britain in the mid 19th century and in 1871 Public Vaccinators were appointed.

There are already many senior members of the medical establishment in Europe and America who want vaccination to be compulsory. You will not be convulsed with shock when I tell you that drug companies which make vaccines would not be averse to their products being made compulsory. I understand that. I would like my books to be made compulsory reading.

Politicians have been persuaded that vaccinating the population at large helps save money. The theory is that if you vaccinate 1,000,000 children against, say, whooping cough (aka pertussis) and, as a result, you prevent 1,000 children getting the disease then the country will avoid the cost of 1,000 parents staying at home for a week or so to look after their child. If one child is permanently brain damaged by the vaccine that is bad luck on the child and his or her parents but, as long as the State can avoid financial responsibility by denying that there is any link between vaccination and brain damage, then it is ahead of the game. In reality, the evidence suggests that even this cold-blooded, steel-hearted philosophy is faulty. The problem is that vaccines are so ineffective and (more important) so dangerous that instead of being an advantage to society as a whole they are a costly disadvantage - though the greater part of those costs tend to be transferred from the State to individual families. (In the heat of their enthusiasms for vaccination your GP and health visitor might have forgotten to tell you all this.)

Despite all this evidence, vaccines for children and adults are compulsory in some countries. In other countries (such as the UK) doctors are given a financial bonus as a reward when they `sell' vaccination to a large proportion of their patients. Doctors write to patients to encourage them to take their children to the surgery for vaccinations not because they've looked at the evidence and know that a vaccine save lives but because they get paid huge fees for giving vaccinations (or telling their nurse to do them) and massive bonuses if they hit the targets they've been given by the Government. Health visitors and nurses bully patients into accepting vaccinations because that's what they are told to do. If they were told to herd everyone into gas chambers they'd do that too. The world is getting scarier by the minute. Fear upon fear upon threat. Nurses and doctors do what they are told and patients suppress their natural scepticism, stand in line, bare their arms and take what is coming to them.

As more and more people become wary about vaccines so it is likely that more and more countries will make vaccination compulsory. This will happen quickly. Massachusetts, in the USA, passed a law whereby the police can break in and give you a flu shot or put you in jail if you refuse.

In an increasing number of countries, parents who refuse to have their children vaccinated are likely to be arrested and to have their children taken away from them. In other countries (such as the UK) doctors are given a financial bonus as a reward when they `sell' vaccinations to a large enough proportion of their patients. I received an e-mail from the Czech Republic asking for permission to translate the material on vaccines from my website because, I was told, vaccination is now compulsory there and no anti-vaccination material is available. Governments are enthusiastic about vaccines because they believe that vaccinations help stop the spread of diseases in a community and therefore save money. When kids have measles their mums stay off work. That costs the economy money. Vaccines are given to minimise disruption and to save money. The authorities are now even talking of giving the rubella vaccine to young boys to help cut the incidence of that disease among pregnant women.

In Britain, recommendations relating to vaccines are made by the Joint Committee on Vaccination and Immunisation which is made up of a variety of people. I would be very surprised if, at any one time, the committee did not include one or more members who were or are linked in some way to drug companies making vaccines. I have been researching vaccination and drug hazards for over 40 years and I have not yet found an official committee on drug use and safety which did not include individuals with drug company links. (I have on occasions in the past found committees which were composed pretty well entirely of individuals who had financial links with drug companies.)

Incidentally, in July 2011 it was announced that the JCVI had `agreed with a call from the UK Vaccine Industry Group to allow manufacturers to submit evidence for effectiveness and cost earlier in the process'. I wonder who will be first to suggest that the two groups merge to save administration costs.

Up until 2009, the JCVI made what it called `recommendations'. But then the Labour Government created a Statutory Instrument amending the Public Health (Control of Diseases) Act 1984, and so now recommendations of the JCVI will in future receive the full support of the Secretary of State for Health. They will, effectively, become law.

Will the JCVI make vaccination compulsory? Well, I suspect that the better question would probably be: `When will the JCVI make vaccination compulsory?' As more and more people become wary about vaccines so it is likely that more and more countries will make vaccination compulsory. In April 2011, it was announced that the General Medical Council in the UK now requires doctors to be: `immunised against common serious communicable diseases where vaccines are available'. I am a registered and licensed general practitioner. I do not intend to have any vaccinations. I invite the GMC to take whatever action they feel appropriate. I will then ask them to produce evidence proving that all available vaccines are both safe and effective. That should be fun.

The Government will try to reduce the size (and cost of the NHS) because they have to save so much money to avoid national bankruptcy that not even the NHS will be immune to cuts. But the cuts won't be enough. And so, the Government's advisers will suggest that it might help to cut costs if the nation became healthier. And that will, of course, mean more laws. It will mean compulsory all sorts of things. It may mean that people who are overweight and who refuse to lose weight may be fined or punished in some other way (possibly by being denied treatment or benefits). But my best bet is that the Government will introduce a compulsory vaccination programme. The drug companies and the doctors (both of whom will make vast amounts of money out of a compulsory vaccination programme) will recommend that all children be vaccinated whether or not their parents approve. This is already happening in some parts of the world and it isn't difficult to find doctors who are eager to promote compulsory vaccination programmes and who threaten to withhold all medical care from unvaccinated patients. Those parents who refuse to have their children vaccinated will have them taken away from them. As Dr Ron Paul, American Presidential Candidate, has pointed out: `When we give Government the power to make medical decisions for us, we, in essence, accept that the State owns our bodies.'

Britain isn't the only country in Europe which is heading for compulsory vaccination. The French, for example, have also started talking about mass vaccination programmes and I have absolutely no doubt that compulsory vaccination is EU policy. And since the EU always gets what it wants, compulsory vaccination will come to be.

One local authority in England has already created secret vaccination centres, stating that it is doing so under `special powers granted to HM Government under the Civil Contingencies Act 2004'. And another NHS Trust has recently sent out letters inviting people to attend for vaccination. The letter states: `It is important that you attend this session. If you are unable to attend, you will need to go to one of the later sessions listed overleaf.'

That sounds to me very much as though the NHS Trust already regards vaccination as compulsory. And a good many doctors would heartily approve. Senior doctors recently suggested not only that vaccination should be compulsory but that children who were not vaccinated should not be allowed into school. Social workers would doubtless be quick (and eager) to take children away from parents who opposed vaccination. I recently received a letter from a British reader telling me that she had been told by her GP that if she wouldn't accept the swine flu vaccination she would never again be allowed to have any prescription drugs. And yet doctors and nurses aren't always quite so keen about being vaccinated themselves. A group of nurses in Washington, USA fought a mandatory vaccine programme. Around 16,000 registered nurses filed a federal lawsuit seeking an injunction to stop the programme designed to force nurses to accept vaccination against flu or to face losing their jobs. Now, why would so many nurses refuse a vaccine?

Why will vaccination become compulsory?

Simple.

As I showed earlier, politicians have been persuaded (by entirely spurious and Statist arguments) that vaccinating the population at large helps save money and benefits the many at the expense of the few.

Drug companies tighten the screw on politicians by threatening to move their industry abroad, to some more congenial environment, if their suggestions are not heeded. And, of course, they hire strong, efficient lobbyists to promote their cause and to ensure that journalists are kept `on message' and that inconvenient truths are ignored.

In my view, the drug industry is made up of nasty companies run by nasty, ruthless people who care nothing whatsoever for people but who care a great deal for money. In many previous books of mine I have exposed the nasty behaviour of the drug industry which likes to describe itself as `ethical' but which is, I believe, rather more contemptible than the Columbian drug barons who sell cocaine but who do not exhibit such nauseating quantities of hypocrisy.

Having considered the available evidence I have come to the conclusion that parents who unquestioningly trust the Government and their doctor to tell them when to have their child vaccinated (and what with) are reckless beyond forgiveness and unfit to care for a child. They would deserve to have their child taken from them if this would not mean putting their child into the hands of the Government and a bunch of drug company indoctrinated doctors.

And any doctor or nurse who vaccinates a child should be locked up as a child abuser.

It seems to me that every day that goes by we get closer to a position where vaccination programmes will be compulsory. We will all be forced, by law, to accept vaccinations whether we want them or not.

If and when vaccination does become compulsory I intend to sign certificates for myself and my wife stating that we cannot be given vaccines for health reasons. I am a registered and licensed general practitioner and unless the General Medical Council removes my name from the register my advice will, I believe, have to be followed. It is my intention to provide such certificates for any readers who may require them. I rather fancy the idea of holding mass anti-vaccination events in halls around the country. The list of contraindications to vaccination can be lengthy (and are, inevitably, always changing) and it shouldn't be too difficult to find a good reason why most people shouldn't be vaccinated on health grounds. If that fails we can always found a new religion which disapproves of vaccination and use the Human Right Act to protect us from the mad jabbers.

## 13. Vaccines, Immunity and Good Health

It is well known that people who are healthy are more resistant to disease. For example, infectious diseases are least likely to affect (and to kill) those who have healthy immune systems.

Sadly, and annoyingly, we still don't know precisely how immunity works and if we still don't know precisely how immunity works, it is difficult to see how can we possibly know exactly how vaccines might work - and what damage they might do. However, this is a potentially embarrassing and inconvenient problem and so it is an issue that is not discussed within the medical establishment.

What we do know is that since vaccines are usually given by injection they by-pass the body's normal defence systems. Inevitably, therefore, vaccination is an extremely unnatural process. (The words `extremely unnatural process' should worry anyone concerned about long term consequences.)

The good news is that we can improve our immunity to disease by eating wisely, by not becoming overweight, by taking regular gentle exercise and by avoiding regular contact with toxins and carcinogens (such as tobacco smoke and the carcinogens in meat). If doctors gave advice on these issues, and explained what is known about the immune system, they could without doubt save many lives. But where's the profit in giving such simple advice? Drug companies can't make any money out of it. And neither can doctors.

That isn't cynicism or scepticism, by the way. It's straightforward, plain, unvarnished, ungarnished truth.

I no longer believe that vaccines have any role to play in the protection of the community or the individual. Vaccines may be profitable but, in my view, they are neither safe nor effective. I prefer to put my trust in building up my immune system.

## 14. Vaccines and Preventive Medicine

I am an enthusiastic supporter of the principle of preventive medicine. It is usually much easier to avoid an illness than it is to treat one.

Vaccination programmes are usually sold to the public as though they are an integral part of a general preventive medicine programme but over the years I have steadily come around to the view that vaccination programmes cannot truly be described as preventive medicine but are, rather, a part of the interventionist approach to medical care.

Proper preventive medicine (persuading people to avoid really bad habits and to live a healthy lifestyle) is always difficult to sell to politicians, doctors and journalists because you cannot see the people who have been saved. Where is the evidence that something has been done? And more important where is the profit? The idea of vaccination, on the other hand, is very easy to sell to people. And it is enormously profitable for drug companies and doctors.

People love vaccination because it promises them an easy way to avoid illness without having to do anything themselves. They want to believe that it works and they want to believe that it is safe. It is for this reason that vaccines against just about everything (including obesity) are being introduced.

Vaccination is the only form of preventive medicine with which doctors and nurses are very well acquainted, and about which they are most enthusiastic. It's just a real pity that the most significant known facts about vaccines are that they can cause brain damage and they can kill. Indeed, the evidence suggests that vaccines kill and injure far more people than the diseases the vaccines are given to protect against. (Remember, if you will, the fact that in

2010 the American Government officially recognised that a total of 2,800 previously perfectly healthy children had been officially killed or injured by vaccination and that they and their parents had received $110 million in damages. Then, ask yourself how many more thousands of children had been unofficially killed or injured. And, finally, remind yourself that before their vaccinations those children were perfectly healthy and that they were being vaccinated against diseases such as measles and mumps.)

Despite the evidence to the contrary, the medical profession seems to have unlimited faith in the power and usefulness of vaccination. A reader of mine who was not feeling well rang his doctor. He was told: `Stay where you are until you're feeling better then pop into the surgery and the nurse will give you a vaccination.' He hadn't even told the receptionist what was wrong with him.

## 15. Vaccinating Children in Developing Countries

Children in developing countries (often poorly fed and forced by circumstances to drink water which is teeming with bacteria and other nasties) are now being vaccinated by teams of workers from rich countries. Vaccination programmes are paid for by large charitable organisations and by Governments. Undoubtedly well-meaning billionaires do it too. For example, an American software billionaire called Bill Gates has apparently donated $10 billion to create new vaccines. If Gates wants to do some good with his money he would surely be better advised to spend it on providing roads, clean water and reliable food supplies for the many oppressed countries where these things are desperately needed. Or he could spend some of his money campaigning against the selfish, imperialist and wicked policies of the American Government - policies which are directly responsible for much of the pain and disease in the developing world. But vaccines sound cutting edge and exciting and dramatic and pictures of aid workers vaccinating small children make good propaganda. Which newspaper or TV station is going to publish pictures of a new water well being dug? Boring.

The people who organise such vaccination programmes, probably think they are doing good. However, I have no doubt at all that they are doing far more harm than good.

On the 13th June 2011 the British Government announced it was going to spend £800,000,000 of the little money the country had left on buying profitable poisons to jab into innocent, starving babies around the world. As far as I could see no one, but no one, in the media questioned the scientific validity of giving money to Global Alliance for Vaccines and Immunisation. The new patronising imperialism is seen as a `good' thing because no one dares to ask the simple questions. Such as: Why?

It has been shown that the Government could do far more good by, for example, providing soap for handwashing but such simple and cost–effective remedies are neglected.

Incidentally, in May 2011, it was announced that a vaccine company was set to join the board of the Global Alliance for Vaccines and Immunisation. Crucell, a company owned by an American healthcare group, makes 60 per cent of its revenue from the Global Alliance for Vaccines and Immunisation and one of its representatives will in future sit on the board. This is, however, apparently of little consequence, for the *Financial Times* has pointed out that 'all members of the board have conflicts'.

As far as journalists are concerned `vaccines are good' and anyone who questions their use can be denounced as a bad, bad person.

It would be nice if the Government used one per cent of the money it is giving to Global Alliance for Vaccines and Immunisation on some original research to find out whether vaccines are safe and effective. But they won't do that. The results might be inconvenient.

## 16. How Effective Is Vaccination?

Between 20 per cent and 50 per cent of individuals who are vaccinated against a disease do not develop a resistance to the disease against which they have been allegedly immunised. In other words up to half of the healthy individuals who are vaccinated (and whose health and lives are therefore put at risk) gain no benefit whatsoever from the vaccination.

In their rush to get to the next patient, doctors and nurses may sometimes forget to mention this.

## 17. Contraindications to Vaccination

Drug companies publish a long list of reasons for not vaccinating patients. Doctors rarely even look at the list, let alone take any notice of it.

Here's the list of contraindications and warnings for one vaccine selected at random: `Acute severe febrile illness. Encephalopathy of unknown aetiology within 7 days after previous vaccination. Progressive neurological disorder, uncontrolled epilepsy or progressive encephalopathy. Severe local or general reaction to a preceding dose of vaccine. History of febrile convulsions, fever, shock or persistent crying within 48 hours of previous vaccination. Guillain-Barre syndrome or brachial neuritis following vaccination.' Those are reasons for not giving one particular vaccine.

Now, imagine the contraindications and possible adverse effects when three or four vaccines are mixed together into a single vaccine cocktail.

## 18. Vaccine Side Effects (Including Brain Damage)

There are doctors and nurses around who deny that vaccines can produce any side effects at all. There are, they claim, no risks whatsoever. Personally, I feel that any doctor who claims that any vaccine, or any drug, does not produce side effects should be enrolled in a reliable space programme and shot into orbit. He or she is too dangerous to practise medicine and far too stupid to be recycled in any useful capacity. But that's just my personal opinion. The medical establishment, and its very best chum the international pharmaceutical industry, would undoubtedly rather see me fired off into space.

When patients fall ill after being vaccinated the doctors who don't believe that vaccines can cause side effects (and who probably also believe that the earth is the centre of the universe) wave aside any link between the two and dismiss the illness as a coincidence. Whatever happens they arbitrarily decide that it is impossible for any side effects to be caused by their beloved and highly profitable vaccines. What many fail to realise is that vaccination damage may occur weeks, months or years after vaccination. By then the time interval between the vaccination and the damage may be so long that no one connects the two.

If these craven, witless apologists for vaccination were proper doctors, in the tradition of Semmelweiss, Snow, Lister and the other gods of medicine, if they cared a twopenny damn about their patients, or if they had any respect for their profession, they would, of course, report every potential side effect to the authorities and allow epidemiologists to decide whether or not specific health problems were, or were not, associated with vaccination. But sadly, I fear, doctors have already decided that vaccination is far too profitable a side-line for them to risk damaging it by finding out the truth. Tragically, many doctors seem to be painfully ignorant about the vaccines they advocate. They do what they are told to do, unquestioningly and unthinkingly, and check their bank balance every month to make sure that the nice, big, fat Government payments have gone through satisfactorily.

The truth is that of all the forms of drugs available vaccines are the crudest and the most unreliable and the most dangerous. (They are also the most profitable but that, of course, is merely a coincidence.) Vaccines can cause brain damage - and can kill. I'm always startled that this should surprise anyone. If you inject potentially toxic substances into small children it seems pretty obvious to me that you will get problems. (If you doubt the effect of toxic substances on the brain remember the last time you saw (and heard) Ozzie Osbourne on television.) The most significant known fact about vaccines is that they can cause brain damage. And they can kill. This isn't theory or supposition. It is fact. And yet potential problems are not properly investigated. For example, doctors have noticed that there is a relationship between vaccination and protracted, inconsolable high-pitched screaming occurring shortly afterwards. This seems to be consistent with a link between vaccination and encephalopathy. This link could be deeply embarrassing for politicians, doctors and drug companies and has not been properly investigated.

Astonishingly, when the American Academy of Paediatrics announced that one in six American children had a developmental disorder and or a behavioural disorder no one mentioned the possibility that vaccines might, just might, be responsible. No one in authority seems to know just why so many American children should be in such poor shape. `It doesn't seem fair,' said one expert. `We look after our children so well. American children have more vaccinations than children in any other country.' Four separate studies have shown that there are higher rates of asthma in fully vaccinated children. Some doctors believe that the epidemic of ADHD (now supposed to be affecting millions of children) could be related to vaccination. If ADHD exists (and there is much doubt about that) then it certainly could be caused by vaccination. And if it is then the children diagnosed with the disease are suffering twice. They are made ill by a vaccine and they are then treated with heavy medication which is, in my view, too dangerous to use as landfill. And then there is autism which I deal with later in this book and which is, when in its most serious form, merely an ill-fitting cover up diagnosis for brain damage.

When it was announced that from autumn 2008, British schoolgirls aged 12 to 13 would be vaccinated against cervical cancer it was estimated that the contract for supplying the vaccine against the human papillomavirus would be worth hundreds of millions of pounds. But when the vaccine was introduced it was already known that it could cause problems.

Here's a list of some of the side effects which may be caused by vaccination. Not all vaccines produce all these side effects, of course. But, on the other hand, this list is by no means complete and there are undoubtedly other side effects which may result from vaccination. Brain damage, paralysis, pain, fever, nausea, dizziness, gastro-intestinal disturbances, lost appetite, restlessness, headache, malaise, pain, allergy reaction, irritability, itching, Bell's Palsy, Guillain-Barré syndrome and seizures are just some of the more serious problems. Just how many side effects and problems are there? It's difficult to say. And how common are side effects? That's also difficult to say. Back in 2007, the US Food and Drug Administration (FDA) detailed 1,637 reports of adverse reactions to the vaccination for human papillomavirus (HPV) including 371 serious reactions and three deaths. Most of the time, however, the authorities (by which I mean the Government and the medical establishment) prefer to sweep the details about vaccine related problems under the carpet rather than to promote them.

Vaccines can even cause symptoms which seem to me to be very similar to the symptoms of the disease they are supposed to prevent. So, for example, the milder of the `side effects' known to be associated with the flu vaccine include: fever, tiredness, muscle aching and headache. Are those not the symptoms of the flu? (Those, by the way, are the manufacturer's list of side effects, not mine.) A complete list of the possible side effects associated with the flu vaccine may also include: asthma, brain swelling, Guillian-Barré syndrome, facial paralysis, damage to eye muscles, damage to the arm and shoulder muscles, bruising, abdominal pain, kidney disorders, hives and anaphylaxis. A study published in the *International Journal of Clinical Investigation* showed that those who have had the flu jab for five years in a row have a ten fold increased risk of developing Alzheimer's disease. Doctors always seem to forget to mention this when pushing their annual (and highly profitable) flu jab campaigns. It is not known whether the flu vaccine can trigger cancer, infertility or other serious health problems. The body's immune system fights cancerous cells and, indeed, some anti-cancer therapies are designed to boost the immune system and to help it fight a developing cancer. Could repeated vaccinations affect the body's susceptibility to cancer? Could repeated vaccinations make the body less able to deal with a developing cancer? Could the constant increase in the incidence of cancer be a result of the enthusiasm for vaccination programmes which has for decades now been inspired by drug companies and maintained by Governments and doctors? Dunno. But I do know that one anti-flu vaccine which was injected into over a million American citizens contained a cancer-causing monkey virus. Some doctors believe that vaccination programmes are causing insulin dependent diabetes mellitus. The suggestion is that the diabetes does not develop for several years after the vaccination. This theory needs investigating.

In 1998, the Pentagon, fearful of germ warfare, began again to vaccinate all military personnel against anthrax. `We were told to shut up and stick your arm out,' says a former female helicopter pilot who stopped menstruating after the first shot and had by the third of the six shot series lost a third of her body weight. As the vaccine's alleged casualties (including six deaths) mounted so soldiers began to refuse it. Around 400 resigned or were court martialled for refusing the vaccine. The irony, of course, was that only the Americans had the capacity to wage biological war. No one should have been surprised by any of the terrible things that happened in the late 1990s. Approximately 25 per cent of soldiers participating in the Gulf War in 1990-1991 were made sick by the anthrax vaccine they were given. (Incidentally, it has been alleged that a component used in that anthrax vaccine was later introduced in one of the swine flu vaccines approved for use in the UK.)

Vaccinations have been linked to a number of other general health problems. It now seems possible, for example, that individuals who receive vaccinations may be more prone to develop allergies (such as asthma), arthritis, eczema and bowel disease (such as Irritable Bowel Syndrome). The explanation - which makes sense to me - is that vaccinations interfere with the immune system and make the recipients more susceptible to disease. The human immune system is a wonderland of protection. It is one of God's great gifts to us. And yet, as I showed in my book *Superbody*, our immune systems are being battered and broken and damned near destroyed by environmental factors largely outside our control. What if vaccines damage the immune system in some way? We know that when the immune system is damaged people become more susceptible to illness. And more likely to die. Just how much damage are vaccines doing? It is possible, and I believe extremely likely, that vaccines damage the human immune system and, as a result, weaken people and make them more likely to fall ill in the future. People with poor immune systems are more susceptible to infectious diseases and more likely to succumb to cancer. Are some vaccines more dangerous than others? How many people die because their immune systems have been damaged by vaccines?

I still have no idea of the answer to any of these (officially) unasked questions. Your doctor doesn't have any answers either. He'll waffle and burble and tell you that the Government says vaccines are wonderful and ask you, with a sneery, knowing smile, if you really think the Government is out to kill your children and he'll tell you I'm a dangerous heretic. But he won't have any answers. And, remember, he gets paid for giving vaccinations.

In 1998, the French Government abandoned its mandatory Hepatitis B vaccine programme for schoolchildren after more than 15,000 lawsuits were filed for brain damage and autoimmune reactions including arthritis, multiple sclerosis and lupus.

In an infant the brain is developing very quickly. During this time infants are given an ever-increasing barrage of vaccinations. You might imagine that dumping all this potentially toxic stuff into a developing body might put a huge strain on the developing immune system. Scientists have not yet looked into this. I find myself constantly puzzled by the failure of other doctors to question what is happening. Who (other than a drug company spokesman) wouldn't expect an infant to show serious signs of distress when deliberately injected with potentially toxic foreign substances? Why shouldn't such injections cause a severe immune response? What, you may wonder, is the effect of squirting all this gunk into babies and small children? I certainly wonder. And, I hope that one or two members or the medical establishment will one day have the wit, and the conscience, to wonder too.

Meanwhile, as we wait for more research work explaining precisely how much damage vaccines do, we should perhaps all remember that the American Government has officially recognised that in the year 2010 `perfectly safe' childhood vaccines officially killed or injured 2,699 children in America. And that, remember, is 2,699 children who were perfectly healthy before they had their vaccinations. Those children, and their families, paid quite a price so that drug companies and doctors could make a great deal of money. We should be aware, too, that there are still many unanswered (and usually unasked) questions about vaccination. For example, we know that vaccines cause neurological damage. And we know that the first symptoms of disease may appear some considerable time after vaccination has taken place. 'Is it possible,' asked my wife, Donna Antoinette, when she had read an early draft of this book, 'that the rise in the incidence of multiple sclerosis (MS) could be a consequence of the increase in childhood vaccination? Could the increase in the number of young women affected by MS be a result of the extra vaccines now given to young girls?' I had to tell her that I have no idea. Moreover, I doubt if any of the gung-ho vaccinators have ever even asked those questions – let alone thought about answering them.

Finally, here is a quote from a former American vaccine researcher: `*If I had a child now, the last thing I would allow is vaccination. I would move out of the State if I had to. I would change the family name. I would disappear. With my family. I'm not saying it would come to that. There are ways to sidestep the system with grace, if you know how to act. There are exemptions you can declare, in every State, based on religious and/or philosophic views. But if push came to shove I would go on the move.*'

Food for thought?

## 19. Are Cot Deaths Caused By Vaccination?

It has been suggested that vaccinations may be the explanation for the mystery problem known as `cot death' (or Sudden Infant Death Syndrome). Children who die of `cot death' tend often to die just after they have received their first vaccinations. What a coincidence. Why hasn't the medical establishment noticed that many of the babies who die of `cot death' often die just days after the recommended dates for childhood vaccinations?

Are so-called `cot deaths' merely another terrible consequence of Government-approved vaccination programmes?

It is interesting to note that when vaccinations were postponed until the 24th month of life in Japan, the incidence of cot death pretty well disappeared. The medical establishment will dismiss this as probably just yet another coincidence.

I'm not so sure.

Until someone proves otherwise I suspect that cot death is just another awful side effect of vaccination. And cot death is now the leading cause of death in children between one month and one year in age.

## 20. Shaken Baby Syndrome and Vaccination

It seems that in cases where parents (and others) have been accused of murdering their children by shaking them, or in some other way abusing them, the real culprit may well have been a vaccine.

Around the world an increasing number of parents have been arrested and charged with injuring or killing their babies. Some of those parents are undoubtedly guilty. But many (and possibly most) are not because in many cases the baby or young child almost certainly died not because he or she was attacked by a parent who had lost control but because his or her brain was damaged by a vaccine or some other medication.

Shaken Baby Syndrome (in which the brain is damaged by a vaccine) is now a very real problem in all societies where vaccines are routinely (and in some countries forcibly) administered. The damage done to the baby or child by the vaccine mimics the damage that would be done if the baby was forcefully shaken.

The problem is that when the police investigate the sudden death of a child, and a pathologist produces a report showing that the child died because of brain damage, the chances are high that one of the parents will be charged with murder. In America this can mean that the misinformed prosecution will call for the death penalty.

A lot of people (Governments, drug companies and the medical establishment) have a powerful, financial interest in suppressing the truth and so naturally, doctors and drug companies deny that vaccines can kill in this or any other way. Compliant journalists believe what they are told and naively print the denials.

The doctors and drug companies cannot, however, deny that brain damage is a well-known possible side effect of vaccination and that brain swelling, intracranial bleeding and other symptoms of `shaken baby syndrome' can all be produced by vaccines. This fact isn't widely known - perhaps because doctors and drug companies would rather that unfortunate parents always took the blame for these deaths.

I'm not saying that all cases of `shaken baby syndrome' are caused by vaccines.

But I do believe that some, or many, of these sad deaths are a consequence of vaccination.

And it would be nice if the authorities would admit the risk and the association so that at least some of the innocent parents who are wrongly convicted of murder might at least have a fair trial.

It doesn't seem a lot to ask.

# 21. Vaccines Contain Much Stuff That You Probably Didn't Know Was There

Vaccines have to be developed using living systems and are usually cultivated in material taken from animals - in cell cultures or in the blood of infected animals. Tissues which have been used include brain tissue from rabbits, kidney tissue from dogs, rabbits and monkeys, protein from fertilised hens' or ducks' eggs and blood from horses or pigs. There are a number of potential problems with creating vaccines in this way and this system can, of course, be dangerous since cell cultures may be contaminated (as was the case with the polio vaccine made with monkey tissue). More recently, some vaccines were prepared using bovine serum and it now appears that during the early 1990s an unknown number of British children received vaccinations which may have been prepared using material from British cattle which could have been infected with BSE. Naturally, no one knows the size of the risk that was taken at the time (though it seems that the British Government was warned of the hazard but chose to ignore the risk). No one is likely to know the size of any problem resulting from this for many years to come. The official position is that we must all hope for the best. In reality, I doubt if anyone will ever do the necessary research to find out how many individuals were adversely affected by contaminated vaccine. If no research is done there won't be any embarrassing results, any adverse publicity affecting vaccination programmes and no successful lawsuits.

Vaccines may contain all sorts of substances in addition to the remnants of the infection against which they are supposed to be providing protection. Other substances found in vaccines include: albumin, formaldehyde, various amino acids, DNA residues, egg protein, gelatine, surfactants, monosodium glutamate and various antibiotics.

In addition, vaccine manufacturers now sometimes use adjuvants - chemicals included to enhance the immune response so that less viral material can be used in each vaccine dose. The alleged benefit is that this enables the manufacture to make the available vaccine go further. When they were introduced, adjuvants were not approved in the USA because their use was untested. However, Britain did not ban the use of the products. Why would anyone want to test a product to see if it was safe? That would be as daft as testing it to see if it worked.

And there are other additives. Antibiotics may be added to dampen down the immune system response. And stabilisers of various kinds may also be included.

Every time something is added to a vaccine the chances of problems developing are increased.

Many vaccines contain thimerosal which contains mercury. Mercury is one of the most toxic substances known to man. This means that when children are vaccinated they are injected with mercury. Vaccines have been made which give more than 50 times the safe amount. Vaccines used in America have not contained mercury since 2001 because it is known that mercury can cause neurological damage. The World Health Organisation has stated that there is no safe level of mercury in the human body. Vaccines may also contain aluminium - which can cause brain damage. Curiously, the European Union demands a ban on barometers which contain mercury (on the grounds that they are dangerous) but allows drug companies to sell vaccines which contain mercury. In what way, I wonder, is it safer to inject mercury into babies than it is to have it in a barometer hanging on the wall?

Inevitably, it is not uncommon for vaccines to contain material which shouldn't be there and which wasn't put there deliberately. Contaminants which have been found in vaccines include: chicken viruses, acanthamoeba, simian cytomegalovirus, simian foamy virus, bird cancer viruses, enzyme inhibitors, duck viruses, dog viruses, rabbit viruses, avian leucosis virus and pestivirus. What harm can these contaminants do? I don't know. I don't think anyone else does either. When companies use tissue from a bird to make a vaccine they have no idea how many germs may be in that tissue. Some vaccines are made with aborted human foetal tissue. For example, part of the original MMR vaccine was taken from cells cultured from an aborted human foetus. Nice to know. Again, no one knows what diseases might be carried in that tissue. Doctors using these vaccinations are practising a form of cannibalism. If you wouldn't eat someone's dead human baby why would you want your child to be injected with tissue from that baby?

In January 2009, contaminated flu virus material was released from a plant in Austria. The error was only discovered because the contaminated product was used in experiments with ferrets. Unexpectedly, the ferrets died. On other occasions medicines have been deliberately contaminated. It would not be impossibly difficult for a determined person to contaminate a vaccine intended for use on millions of people.

## 22. Is Autism Caused By Vaccination?

The number of children diagnosed as suffering from autism has rocketed just as the number of children being vaccinated has risen. This isn't just true of the UK; it's true of all countries where children are vaccinated. I have for many years believed (and argued) that epidemiologically and logically all varieties of autism (including such brands as Asperger's) are nothing more than vaccine damage. Where's the evidence? Well, there's a startling absence of research but in the USA a huge medical practice of paediatricians with 30,000 child patients do not vaccinate their patients at all. They have no patients with autism. In the old days such an observation (known as epidemiological research) was regarded as valuable. Today, bizarrely, it is dismissed as irrelevant.

Some patients with autism are severely damaged and some are lightly damaged. Only a complete fool (or someone more enthusiastic about money than truth) would deny that there might be a link. But when a research project was set up to investigate any link between vaccination and autism drug companies applied to a court for an injunction to stop the research. Now, why would they do that?

Here are seven incontrovertible facts.

Fact one: Autism is (in its more serious forms) a disorder which involves brain damage.

Fact two: Vaccines cause brain damage. (If vaccines are known to cause brain damage isn't it logical to assume that they may also cause the disease which is known as autism but which would, I believe, be more properly and honestly known as vaccine brain damage? I suspect that the children currently being diagnosed as `autistic' are actually suffering from various levels of brain damage caused by vaccines - and should have been awarded damages by drug companies, doctors and the Government.)

Fact three: The incidence of autism has rocketed as the number of vaccinations being given has also rocketed. There's a surprising correlation between the two. If someone noticed a statistical correlation between the number of people sucking humbugs and the number of people losing their teeth I bet you a devalued pound to a devalued penny that teams of highly paid medical scientists would start investigating. (The humbug manufacturers would complain but I doubt if they have as much clout as the international pharmaceutical industry.) Once rare (in the 1990s it was generally accepted that autism affected no more than 4 or 5 people in every 10,000), it is now officially claimed that autism affects more than 100 in every 10,000 children in Britain. (Some experts claim that the real figure is much higher than this.) Figures from around the world show that the incidence of autism is rising in all developed countries - just as the number of vaccinations given is rising. None of this proves that vaccines cause autism but how anyone can simply deny the possibility of a link between vaccination and autism is quite beyond me. The epidemiological evidence is overwhelming.

Fact four: Children who suffer from brain damage after vaccination are numbed and need a good deal of stimulation. They respond well to flashing lights, colours and movement. Exactly the same thing happens with children suffering from severe autism.

Fact five: Some so-called experts claim that autism is caused by environmental pollution. Curiously, these `experts' do not believe that injecting foreign matter into small children is pollution.

Fact six: A number of parents have reported that their autistic children responded particularly badly when they were given their childhood vaccinations. From the evidence reported to me I believe that if children scream a good deal after vaccination, or are unusually quiet, or show other unusual signs, then there is, I believe, a real chance that they will develop autism.

Fact Seven: The American Government has reportedly accepted that vaccines may cause autism.

I believe, and have believed for many years, that autism is caused by vaccination. I believe that the evidence (including the epidemiological evidence) supports this hypothesis. I suspect that some children have a hereditary susceptibility and respond badly to vaccination. And if vaccines are known to cause brain damage isn't it logical to assume that they can also cause autism? Isn't it logical to at least want to do some pretty high-powered research to find the nature of the link?

Part of the problem is that there isn't really any clear way to define autism. It is a ragbag diagnosis used to describe a whole range of symptoms - ranging from severe brain damage to relatively mild behavioural problems. Many doctors now agree with me that severe autism is simply vaccine produced brain damage while very mild autism may merely be an excuse to be used when a child doesn't do as well as its parents expected. In those circumstances the diagnosis provides a social excuse for academic failure.

The word autism is used, like the word cancer, as an umbrella term for a range of different problems. Patients with autism are said to have development disorders which affect their ability to interact socially and to communicate with other people though this is a fairly recent interpretation and the word now seems to be used as a catch-all for a whole range of problems. (In one medical dictionary on my shelf autism is defined as `morbid self-absorption' which hardly fits the range of symptoms seen.) These days, I suspect that the word is used more as a dustbin word rather than an umbrella word. It helps the profession appear to know what is the matter when they don't and, at the same time, it enables them to avoid taking any responsibility for what has happened. The word is used to describe almost any symptoms which doctors cannot explain.

Social workers and other professional morons play the game because it enables them to build well-funded empires around the `care' of autistic patients. For governments it is, of course, a lot cheaper to provide a modest amount of `care' for autistic patients than to acknowledge that these children have been made ill by the official vaccination policy, and should have been provided with vast amounts of compensation. Every day that vaccination programmes continue makes it ever more unlikely that governments will ever accept that there is any association between the two.

Doctors and drug companies and politicians much prefer to talk about autism rather than brain damage because the former suggests a natural disease while the latter suggests that there may be an external cause. Innocent and desperate parents collude with this nonsense because they prefer to describe their children as autistic than as brain damaged.

Those who oppose the conclusion that vaccination causes brain damage which is in turn often mislabelled as autism sometimes claim that the recorded incidence of autism is going up because doctors are better at making the diagnosis. This is patent nonsense for which there is no scientific evidence. (It is, I must point out, also possible that the incidence of autism is going up for the same reason that the incidence of other fashionable pseudo diseases such as ADHD is going up. They may all be rising because they are fashionable and popular diseases which suit the personal and political motives of various groups of people - particularly parents who are looking for an appropriate label to stick on their child. Certainly, the list of symptoms said to be associated with autism is now increasing so rapidly that it will soon be easier to diagnose someone as *not* suffering from the disorder.)

I believe that autism was devised so that drug companies could avoid the embarrassment of seeing children described as vaccine damaged. Once the new disease had been invented, drug companies started to sell treatments for this newly created and non-existent disease. You have to admire their marketing brilliance.

The drug companies (and the doctors, hospitals and politicians who support them) all claim that there is no link between autism and vaccination. (But then they would, wouldn't they?). They claim that there is no convincing scientific evidence proving a link between the two. On the other hand there is no convincing scientific evidence disproving a link between vaccination and autism. The one scientific paper I've been able to find which claims to disprove the link between autism and vaccination was written by a group who worked for the Government in Denmark. One of the researchers involved has reportedly been charged with stealing more than $1 million in autism research money from the Centers for Disease Control and Prevention in Atlanta, USA.

In answer to those who still claim that there is no link between vaccination and autism I would again remind readers that the US Health Departments National Vaccine Injury Compensation Programme has reportedly accepted that hundreds of children have officially developed autism after vaccination. That goes quite a long way towards proving that I'm right and the vaccine supporters are wrong.

## 23. Has Your Dinner Been Vaccinated?

Those who eat meat should be aware that cattle (and other animals reared for slaughter) are regularly vaccinated. The meat that is taken from those animals may, therefore, contain vaccine residues in addition to hormones, antibiotics and other drugs. Today, even some farmed fish are individually vaccinated against infections that might damage profits.

## 24. Lawsuits, Damages and Vaccination

The drug companies very rarely lose lawsuits relating to drug or vaccine damage. There are several reasons for this. First, drug companies and doctors tend to stick together, to protect each other's financial interests. The drug companies know that if they lose one lawsuit they will find themselves fighting many more - so they fight very hard. Drug companies have almost bottomless pits of money at their disposal. And they are not averse to warning litigants that if they go ahead, and lose, their homes may be at risk. Another problem is that there is very little scientific evidence relating to the safety of drugs or vaccines and so little published material available for litigants to use. And few doctors are prepared to risk their careers by giving evidence against colleagues or drug companies. One doctor who did give evidence in court found herself fighting for her career before the GMC - because she dared talk honestly about vaccines and vaccination.

It is always difficult to prove that X happened because of Y. For many years the tobacco companies successfully argued that smoking cigarettes had no connection to lung cancer and today the food companies still argue that meat does not cause cancer, even though the evidence proving that the link exists is overwhelming. Similarly, the drug companies rely on the absence of any evidence proving that vaccines cause serious problems. And, finally, the Government never openly admits that vaccines cause problems. And they never will admit this. There are instances where thousands of patients have developed bad effects after vaccination but nothing has happened because the authorities always exonerate vaccines. They always find a way to rule out a link between the vaccine and any ensuing health problem and, as usual, the reason is financial: if the Government admitted that a vaccine caused many health problems then it would be liable to huge damages. What sort of damages? Think of a number and then see how many noughts you can cram after it on a cheque. Nevertheless, as I pointed out in the section on whooping cough vaccination, the British Government has, over the years, already paid out compensation to the parents of many hundreds of children who were brain damaged by the whooping cough vaccine. Some parents who accepted damages in the early years were given £10,000. Later the sum was raised to £20,000. You may not have heard about this. It was done very quietly.

Things are much the same in other countries. The US Secretary of State for Health and Human Services signed a decree granting vaccine makers total legal immunity from any lawsuits that result from any new swine flu vaccine, and the US Government gave $7 billion to ensure that the vaccine was made available quickly and in quantities that would make it possible to carry out mass vaccinations. Naturally, speeding up the whole programme meant that it could be done without boring and 'unnecessary' safety tests beforehand.

Occasionally, brave and persistent parents have won damages against drug companies. For example, in 1992, the Irish Supreme Court found in favour of Margaret Best who sued Wellcome, the maker of a vaccine against whooping cough, on behalf of her son Kenneth Best who had the mental age of a 12-month-old baby. Following a retrial to determine compensation, Kenneth Best was awarded £2.75 million compensation. Sadly, he was 23-years-old at the time so it seems fair to assume that the battle for compensation had taken his courageous and determined mother more than two decades.

This was, however, an exceptional case. Because drug companies rarely accept responsibility for illness caused by the drugs and vaccines they make (and because most parents quite understandably give up the struggle for drug company compensation) families and taxpayers usually end up paying all the bills for the care of vaccine damaged individuals.

## 25. The Companies Which Make Vaccines (And Which Make a Lot of Money

## Out of Them)

Drug companies have for years recognised that their biggest profits will come from treatments devised for chronic illnesses. The advantage here is that these drugs will need to be taken for years - in many cases until a patient dies. Drug companies have also recognised that they make most money when they find a treatment that will be required by a large proportion of the population in a rich country. It is for this reason that drug companies spend so much time and money developing `treatments' for psychiatric problems, high blood pressure,  heart disease, arthritis, thrombosis, osteoporosis, pain relief, high cholesterol, obesity, impotence and baldness.

Vaccines, however, are better than all of these. Vaccines are the answer to a prayer for drug companies. Vaccines are the perfect product. They can be sold for high prices. They can be given to everyone. And they can be given every year. They can be sold in developed countries. And they can be sold in developing countries. Governments can be persuaded to buy them in huge quantities - at top prices. Philanthropists will buy them by the planeload to distribute to doctors in countries where fresh water and enough food to eat are as rare as £1,000 designer handbags. Brilliant.

The result is that drug companies make huge amounts of money out of selling vaccines. And the establishment has fiddled the evidence, and denied or suppressed the inconvenient truths, in order to promote the official point of view. In Britain I have been banned from speaking to doctors. Debates about vaccination are unknown.

The global vaccine market reached $21 billion in 2010 and is growing at a rate of 16.5 per cent. Back in 2006 the market was worth $11.42 billion. Drug companies are constantly producing new products. There are vaccines for children, vaccines for travellers and vaccines for old people. Governments stockpile the damned things `in case of emergency'.

The whole business of vaccinating people is so hugely profitable (largely because it is something that doesn't rely on finding a large number of sick people but also because it is something that can be done on a regular basis) that drug companies, having almost saturated the `vaccinating-children' market are moving heavily into adult vaccines. There is, for example, a vaccine planned to prevent atherosclerosis. I suspect that doctors will claim that this will enable people to keep eating a bad diet and yet avoid heart attacks. It is, of course, fairly easy to prevent the problem by eating wisely but, encouraged by the National Health Service (NHS), most people still prefer to avoid ill health without inconveniencing themselves.

Here's a clue as to the profit to be made out of vaccines. In April 2010, the British Government announced that it had cancelled contracts with a big drug company for 90 million doses of swine flu vaccine. Around 5.5 million people (most of them health workers) had already been vaccinated but the NHS had 30 million unused vaccines left over. Those, said the politicians, would go unused at a cost of £150 million.

Why did they buy so much of the damned stuff? They gave vaccines to 5.5 million people, threw away 30 million vaccines and cancelled a contract for another 90 million vaccines.

Were they planning to invade Europe and vaccinate the French too? Or are there more illegal immigrants in Britain than anyone has previously dared admit?

Now, here's a contrary thought.

Is it remotely possible that the drug industry as a whole could want to make people ill?

The industry does, after all, have a vested interest in making people ill and keeping them that way - so that it can sell them more drugs. Look at it this way: a healthy population would result in the collapse of the international pharmaceutical industry.

Are the ruthless men and women who run this industry determined to keep making vast amounts of money, whatever it takes, or are they determined to damage their profits and, in the end, put themselves out of business by making people healthy?

Simple question.

And I think I know the answer.

I can't leave the subject of drug companies without mentioning the fact that these days they have an enormous amount of influence over the medical profession, the media and just about anyone else likely to be a potential nuisance. It is pretty well known, I think, that doctors are constantly bribed by drug companies (free meals, free travel, free gifts) but journalists are frequently bribed too (`Would you please write an article for our in-house magazine? We can pay you £3,000 for 100 words. Would that be acceptable?').

After my first book, *The Medicine Men*, was published in 1975 a drug company asked if they could sponsor me. They wanted to pay me to give some lectures. I was astonished and declined the offer. (*The Medicine Men* was an attack on the medical profession's close links with the pharmaceutical industry and an analysis of the many ways that the drug company promotes its dangerous products.) Even today I still receive a constant stream of requests from individuals and organisations wanting to advertise on my website. I turn them all down (even though the money would undoubtedly more than pay the costs of running the site) because even if I know that the advertising money won't buy my views (or my silence) some people might worry that it could. Perception is everything.

I mention all this because the drug companies never stop looking for ways to influence the view the world has of what they do, and they have, in recent years, made a concerted effort to create strong links with societies representing patients' interests.

Organisations which are created and run for the benefit of patients usually start small - and are administered either by a patient or a relative or friend. But some organisations grow large - very large - and they often do this by obtaining grants and financial support from large companies. Drug companies are often particularly keen to help such organisations - though my experience of drug companies makes me feel sceptical about this being an entirely altruistic gesture. Why would a drug company give its shareholders' money to an organisation whose members include some who are critical of the industry?

For example, at the end of March 2007, I noticed that the National Autistic Society had a drug company among its supporters. I sent the following letter to Society.

`I see that a drug company which makes MMR vaccine is one of your financial supporters (and has been since 2003). I understand that the company has, for example, paid for mailing over 4,000 GP surgeries with information about autism. Since there is a huge debate ongoing about whether or not autism is caused by the MMR vaccine I would be interested to hear the society's explanation for accepting this funding. Do you not feel that by accepting money from GlaxoSmithKline you are abandoning your independence, your reputation and your value to autistic patients and their carers? I ask these questions as a medical author as well as a registered general practitioner.'

On the 16th April 2007 I received a reply from Benet Middleton, the society's Director of Communications. Here's the reply:

`The question of who to accept funding from is often a difficult issue for all charities, not just the NAS. On the one hand we have to be aware of the issues you raise around reputation and independence and on the other we have to ensure that we generate the income required to provide the support, advice, advocacy and awareness raising that are so vitally needed.'

`Our Board of Trustees adopted a stance that we would not work with any company that acted illegally or acted in contravention to our charitable objectives, in part to reflect that everyone has their own personal ethics and views and it would be impossible to act on all of these. However, in addition we will not enter into partnerships that will have a detrimental effect on people with autism or our reputation.'

`In this case we have accepted money from GSK for a number of small projects, including a GP mailing to raise awareness of autism last year. None of these projects have had any link to anything we have said on the MMR vaccine and GSK have never raised this topic with us. Furthermore, the overall funding to date amounts to such a tiny *percentage of our income that it could not possibly influence our position on this topic when stacked up against the support we receive from people living with autism.'*

Here is my reply:

*`The National Autistic Society isn't alone.*

*Many large and successful charities and organisations set up to help people with specific health problems, accept money from drug companies. It is no surprise that drug companies usually fund organisations which deal with problems appropriate to their products. But, not being entirely stupid, the drug companies never bring up the important issues in any direct way. The fact is, however, that they know that a charity which takes money from a drug company will be compromised and that whatever the charity says will be tainted. Do you honestly believe that the National Autistic Society can now ever produce any worthwhile contribution to the debate on the link between vaccination and autism?*

*Many people (me included) believe that many or even most cases of autism are a result of brain damage caused by vaccination. For the National Autistic Society to accept money from a drug company which produces a vaccine which has been linked to autism in this way seems to me to be extraordinarily immoral.*

*The Society seems to be claiming that it hasn't accepted very much money from GlaxoSmithKline and that it is not, therefore, compromised by this association.*

*So, how much money will GlaxoSmithKline have to give before the National Autistic Society is compromised by the association? How many other drug companies contribute to the Society?*

*(I note, incidentally, that in your letter you refer not to GlaxoSmithKline (the name of the drug company) but simply to GSK - as though not printing out the full name of the company will somehow make the link less embarrassing.)*

*Personally, I feel that a hooker who charges £5 for sex is no less a hooker than a hooker who charges £1,000.*

*This correspondence will appear on my website and in a forthcoming book.'*

I didn't hear from them again.

## 26. Doctors Have Been Bought

Could it be possible that doctors don't search for the truth about vaccines and vaccination programmes because the medical profession has been bought?

The fact is that drug companies aren't the only ones to profit from vaccines. Doctors make large amounts of money from vaccines too. General practitioners (GPs) receive chunky fees for giving vaccines and receive massive bonuses if they can persuade/blackmail/pressurise enough of their patients to have vaccinations. This really is appalling and I fear that GPs lost their final scrap of integrity on the day when they agreed to accept bribe money if they managed to vaccinate enough of the patients they were already being paid to look after. I'm old-fashioned enough to believe that this sort of cold-hearted, conveyor belt, bonus-ridden philosophy is better suited to the manufacture of motor car parts than the practise of medicine. The current system, whereby GPs are paid according to the number of people they vaccinate, is appalling and is nothing more than bribery and corruption. The State is doing the bribing and corrupting. And doctors are the ones who have been bribed and corrupted. The whole idea of giving doctors a bonus according to the number of patients they vaccinate is a bizarre one. Doctors don't get paid more if they prescribe tons of antibiotics or if they refer an officially acceptable percentage of their female patients for hysterectomies.

Only doctors who are very stupid, or ill-informed, do not understand that vaccines are potentially dangerous, inadequately tested and often ineffective. Sadly, it seems that there are far more stupid and ill-informed GPs around than there really ought to be and giving doctors a financial incentive to perform a particular medical procedure has doubtless tilted the balance and persuaded doctors to ignore the hazards. It is a grossly unethical practice and I am appalled both that doctors don't seem to care much about this and that the General Medical Council sees nothing wrong with it.

The tragedy is that I have absolutely no doubt whatsoever that the financial incentive encourages doctors to vaccinate without considering all the possible dangers and complications. The fact that doctors are bribed to vaccinate might suggest to some that the authorities *need* to bribe doctors in order to persuade them to get busy vaccinating. It seems reasonable to assume that if doctors really believed in vaccination they would do it anyway - without the bribes.

It is not unknown for doctors to throw patients off their lists because they won't accept vaccinations - because this affects the GP's earnings. One journalist who interviewed me told me, indignantly, that his own GP had threatened to have his family removed from the GP's list of NHS patients if he would not allow his children to be vaccinated.

And all this goes on in considerable secrecy. How many doctors tell their patients that the Government pays GPs an extra £50,000 a year each, on top of the more than adequate wage of £100,000 to £120,000, which they receive for a basic 40 hour week with no night calls, no weekend duty and no bank holidays, to push their patients into accepting vaccinations? Not many, I suspect, though I believe that those who don't should be serving time for fraud.

Vaccinations are a constant bonanza time for doctors. The basic deal sounds good enough. GPs receive fees from the NHS for giving vaccines and bonus fees for persuading enough of their patients to be vaccinated. But that's not the half of it. The bonanza is even better than that. GPs tell their administrative staff (salaries largely paid for by taxpayers) to order the vaccines and instruct their nurses (whose salaries are also largely or wholly paid for by the taxpayers) to give the vaccinations. All the GP has to do is take time out at the end of a game of golf to ring her accountant to see how much money she has made during a morning of heavy absentee jabbing. A nurse does the jabbing. A clerk fills in the claim form. The doctor just spends the money. Has money ever been earned so easily? Every vaccination GPs give (or authorise) is another nice noise in the cash register. And epidemics produce a bonus bonus. In the autumn of 2009, GPs were demanding a fee of £7.51 to give a swine flu vaccination. Since each patient needed two jabs that meant that each GP stood to earn around £27,000 from giving vaccinations against swine flu. (And, remember, most would tell their practice nurse to give the vaccination and instruct a practice clerk to fill in the claim forms, so they wouldn't have to do anything themselves. So that's a very pleasant £27,000 for doing absolutely bugger all.) With 33,000 GPs in the country, giving the swine flu jabs would have added just under £900 million to the NHS bill.

No wonder there are so many BMW and Mercedes motor cars on the roads these days.

The sad truth is that the enormous and rich vaccine industry, and the Government, have bought the medical profession, lock stock and syringe barrel. GPs, once members of a proud and distinguished profession, a profession which gave the world a seemingly endless series of medical giants, have been reduced to snivelling, whining needle-men for the drug industry; hand-maidens to an industry which cares nothing for people but everything for profits. In my first book, *The Medicine Men*, I wrote that a profession which exists to do the bidding of an industry is no longer a profession. Boy, was I right about that. Doctors have lost their way. The drug industry has done it cleverly, of course. GPs receive massive bonus payments for vaccinating patients not from the drug industry directly but from the Government.

The bribery system works smoothly and well. A GP who jabs enough patients gets a thumping great wodge of cash. A GP who is questioning and discerning will be punished by being paid less. And so the vast majority of GPs, no longer professionals but now just bought slaves, do as they are damned well told.   What a disgrace it is that most know nothing about the dangers of the damned vaccines they so happily jab into patients' arms. And, remember, most don't even do the dirty work themselves. It's far more profitable to tell a Government subsidised hand-maiden to do the work.

The Government will even provide propaganda witches (called health visitors) to chase the patients and the parents who don't turn up to be jabbed. And from time to time, whenever doctors seem to be having difficulty bullying enough patients to accept vaccinations, the Government will do a little deliberate but essential scaring. In attempts to persuade parents to have their children vaccinated against measles, Governments and doctors around the world have thought up an apparently unending - and hysterical - series of scare campaigns. Now that there is a vaccine against it, measles has, by a strange coincidence, stopped being an annoying childhood disease and has, instead, become a deadly killer. Many infectious diseases come in cycles. When a disease is at a high point in its cycle the authorities (egged on by doctors and drug companies) frighten citizens into agreeing to be vaccinated. And when a disease is at a low point in its natural cycle it is vaccination programmes which get the credit.

Scares invariably often consist of claiming that a major epidemic is just around the corner and that only vaccination can offer protection. I have lost count of the number of whooping cough epidemics which Governments have wrongly forecast. Were those official advisors merely incompetent or were they deliberately lying to help boost vaccine uptake and increase drug company profits?

It is difficult to avoid the suspicion that the authorities regularly, and ruthlessly, issue scare warnings in order to frighten people into having the relevant jab.

Now that there are vaccines against all sorts of non-deadly diseases, and children are being vaccinated against diseases such as mumps and measles which were traditionally regarded as inconvenient rather than deadly, these traditional diseases have to be upgraded from `minor childhood disease' to `serious killer'. The plain fact is that in the UK the death rate from measles, for example, had dropped dramatically decades before the vaccine was introduced. It is interesting to note that today, despite (or, dare I say it, perhaps even because of) the widespread use of the vaccine, the incidence of measles has, in some recent years, risen.

Question the whole damned sordid business of vaccination and these ill-educated propagandists (who know nothing about the risks of the toxic mixtures they are promoting) will accuse you of being a flat-earther or a Luddite.

Sadly, tragically, most doctors working for the NHS long ago lost any sense of right or wrong. They long ago lost the passions and beliefs and yearnings that (hopefully) took them into medicine. Today, the lives of the vast majority of practising doctors are driven by a potent and destructive (and distinctly patient-unfriendly) mixture of ambition and greed and denial. There are very few doctors in practice today who want to save the world, or even change it very much. Their aims are selfish and personal. A bigger house, a faster car, shorter working hours and longer holidays.

The bottom line is that NHS GPs have no bloody right to comment on vaccinations. Ever. They are interested parties. A GP's remarks about vaccination are as valuable as those of a drug company spokesman. And yet it has become increasingly common for doctors to complain (publicly) that not enough people are being vaccinated. The vocal doctors involved never mention that they get paid for giving vaccines and therefore have a financial interest in promoting vaccination.

It is important to understand that most of the people who support vaccination are either paid by the drug industry or they obtain their information from people who are paid by the drug industry or, in some other way, they have a vested interest in promoting vaccination. Sadly, GPs have put themselves among the group who have a financial interest in promoting vaccination. General Practice is now no longer a profession; it is a business. GPs who put pressure on patients to have vaccinations, or refuse to treat those who object to vaccination, are, of course, taking purely commercial decisions. If the percentage of patients on their lists who haven't been vaccinated gets too high then the GPs lose out on one of their cash bonuses.

On the other hand, of course, all the people who oppose vaccination do so because they care for children and are worried about the dangers associated with vaccines.

In the same way that the Government has bribed GPs to vaccinate so the Government has, I believe, been bribed, bullied and conned by the drug companies. It has been a brilliant commercial coup. I don't blame the drug companies for manipulating the market, of course. It's what they do. And I don't blame the politicians; they're selfish, uncaring, venal and stupid. But I do blame the GPs. They've sold their honour and integrity and professional birthright and allowed themselves to be bribed into prescribing a specific group of products for personal financial advantage.

There are a thousand things to be angry about.

Doctors often claim that parents who refuse to have their children vaccinated are `bad parents'. Surely it is the parents who allow their children to be injected with a toxic substance, without knowing the truth about what is happening and what is likely to happen, who are bad parents?

Doctors often tell parents that if they don't allow their children to be vaccinated they are allowing their own views to endanger their child's health. Doctors blackmail and pressure patients into accepting vaccination. In some areas children have been taken away from parents who refused vaccination.

How many of those bullying doctors are honest enough to say: `If you don't have your damned kid vaccinated I won't be able to buy my wife a new Mercedes this year?'

It would be nice if doctors provided patients with information instead of simply bullying them. The medical profession's attitude towards vaccination is craven and shameful. I think the worst thing about the medical profession's attitude is that it is motivated by nothing more complicated than simple greed. The doctors who try to make parents feel guilty for caring enough about their children to want more information about vaccination never admit that they themselves have been bribed and bought to promote vaccination. The bottom line is that medical profession, paid by the jab, heavily incentivised to jab, jab and jab again, is giving vaccines which can kill and cause serious, permanent illness, in order to try to protect against diseases which are often relatively trivial or rare and which are unlikely to kill or cause permanent damage. From the evidence I've been able to find I am convinced that the vaccines are doing far more harm than the diseases against which they are supposed to protect. This is patent lunacy. It is also a medical evil of unprecedented horror.

Everyone who has seriously considered the evidence realises that vaccination is far too dangerous and ineffective to be supported. But, sadly, most doctors and nurses no longer think for themselves and are quite incapable of studying original evidence. Today's vaccine promotion is as dishonest as cigarette advertising was in the 1950s and 1960s. The difference is that the cigarette advertisements were stopped by pressure from doctors whereas the vaccine promotion is endorsed by doctors. It is clear that the cigarette industry simply wasn't clever enough to buy the medical profession. And they could have done it so easily. If they had paid doctors healthy fees to hand out cigarettes and to endorse smoking as a health aid, the Government warnings would have never been introduced and the tobacco industry would today be as rich and as prosperous as the global pharmaceutical industry.

I cannot stress enough how important it is to remember that GPs who put pressure on patients to have vaccinations, or who refuse to treat those who object to vaccination, are, of course, taking purely commercial decisions. If the percentage of unvaccinated patients on their lists rises too high then GPs lose out on one of their cash bonuses. GPs, once proud and independent physicians, are now nothing more than paid-for marketing hacks; hired to flog profitable vaccines. (On the other hand, of course, all the people who oppose vaccination do so because they care for children and are worried about the dangers associated with vaccines.)

I should point out that it isn't just GPs who have been bought. It is crucial to remember that the vast majority of people who support vaccination are either paid by the drug industry or they obtain their information from people who are paid by the drug industry or, in some other way, they have a vested interest in promoting vaccination. Nurses, health visitors, journalists and politicians obviously fit into these categories. On the other hand, there are a good many people around who have spent their own time and money on trying to tell the truth about vaccines.

What a terrible thing it is that vaccination is promoted by people who make money out of it and opposed by people who gain nothing and often lose much through their honest opposition. How terrible it is that the happy jabbers in our surgeries and consulting rooms are so blind to the danger of what they are doing. As the writer Upton Sinclair once wrote: `It is difficult to get a man to understand something if his salary depends on his not understanding it.' And before him Adam Smith wrote: `People of the same trade seldom meet together, even for merriment and diversion, but the conversation ends in a conspiracy against the public, or in some contrivance to raise prices.'

How sad it is that doctors have sold themselves, and now conspire against the people they have sworn to protect.


## 27. How the Truth Is Suppressed


These days doctors only get to read and hear what the drug industry wants them to read and hear. Anything controversial, anything questioning the status quo, must be suppressed.

A year or two ago I was invited to speak at a new conference in London. The conference was, I was told, intended to tackle the subject of medication errors and adverse reactions to prescribed drugs. The company organising the conference was called PasTest. `For over 30 years PasTest has been providing medical education to professionals within the NHS,' they told me. `Building on our commitment to quality in medical and healthcare education, PasTest is creating a range of healthcare events which focus on the professional development of clinicians and managers who are working together to deliver healthcare services for the UK. Our aim is to provide a means for those who are in a position to improve services on both national and regional levels. The topics covered by our conferences are embraced within policy, best practice, case study, clinical management and evidence based practice. PasTest endeavours to source the best speakers who will engage audiences with balanced, relevant and thought-provoking programmes. PasTest has proven in the past that by using thorough investigative research and keeping up-to-date with advances in healthcare and medical practice, a premium educational event can be achieved.'

That's what they said.

Sounds wonderful, I thought (in one of my more naive moments).

Iatrogenesis (doctor induced disease) is something of a speciality of mine. I have written numerous books and articles on the subject. My campaigns have resulted in more drugs being banned or controlled than anyone else's.

In addition to my speaking at the conference the organisers wanted me to help them decide on the final programme. I thought the conference was an important one and would give me a good opportunity to tell NHS staff the truth. I signed a contract.

PasTest wrote to confirm my appointment as a consultant and speaker for the PasTest Conference Division. And then there was silence. My office repeatedly asked for details of when and where the conference was being held.

Silence.

Eventually a programme for the event appeared on the Internet. Curiously, my name was not on the list of speakers.

Here is part of the blurb promoting the conference:

`Against a background of increasing media coverage into the number of UK patients who are either becoming ill or dying due to adverse reactions to medication our conference aims to explain the current strategies to avoid Adverse Drug reactions and what can be done to educate patients.'

Putting the blame on patients for problems caused by prescription drugs is brilliant. Most drug related problems are caused by the stupidity of doctors not the ignorance of patients. If the aim is to educate patients on how best to avoid prescription drug problems the advice would be simple: `Don't trust doctors.'

The promotion for the conference claims that `It is estimated errors in medication...account for 4 per cent of hospital bed capacity.' And that prescription drug problems `reportedly kill up to 10,000 people a year in the UK'. As I would have shown (had I not been banned from the conference) these figures are absurdly low.

The list of speakers included a variety of people I had never heard of including one speaker representing The Association of the British Pharmaceutical Industry and another representing the Medicines and Healthcare Products Regulatory Agency.

Delegates representing the NHS were expected to pay £250 plus VAT (□£293.75) to attend the event. Delegates whose Trust would be funding the cost were asked to apply for a Health Authority Approval form.

So why was I apparently banned from this conference?

This is what PasTest said when we asked them: `certain parties felt that he (Vernon Coleman) was too controversial to speak and as a result would not attend.'

Could that `certain parties', I wonder, be the drug industry? Is the drug industry now deciding whom they will allow to speak to doctors and NHS staff on the problems caused by prescription drugs? If I was banned at the behest of the drug industry do NHS bosses know that people attending such conferences will only hear speakers approved by the drug industry and that speakers telling the truth will be banned? (I think it is safe to assume that I won't be invited to speak at any more conferences for NHS staff.)

If I was banned at the behest of the medical profession why are doctors frightened of the truth?

I could not, of course, be banned by the NHS itself. Why would the NHS not want its employees to know the truth about drug related problems?

Why are people who had me banned so frightened of what I would say? It can surely only be because they know that I would have caused embarrassment by telling the truth.

The scary bottom line is that the NHS paid to send delegates to a conference where someone representing the drug industry spoke to them on drug safety. But I was banned. The truth was uninvited.

Details of the ban were sent to every national and major local newspaper in Britain. None reported it.

The question is this: If doctors or drug companies believe I am wrong why don't they let me speak and then explain why I am wrong?

The unavoidable answer is that they know my criticisms of the profession and the industry are accurate and unanswerable.

What happened with PasTest is by no means unusual. All sorts of strange people (mainly politicians and administrators) have taken control of medical care these days; their brains are uncluttered with scientific stuff and they `know best'. Vaccination is now a political issue rather than a scientific issue. Facts are just a damned nuisance that get in the way and about as welcome as hot dog vendors at a meeting of vegetarians.

When the London Assembly (in reality the best known EU Regional Assembly in England) invited members of the public to send in thoughts on vaccination for their `rapporteurship' I sent them a copy of my book *Coleman's Laws*, which contains a lengthy medical explanation of why vaccination is irresponsible and dangerous and a significant cause of illness. An administration officer for the London Assembly wrote to thank me for my views which would, I was assured, be included in their analysis of evidence for the report.

However, there was no mention of any of my evidence in their report and the details of the evidence I had submitted did not appear in the list of references included at the back of the report. I was not surprised by this. Nor was I surprised to see that the report followed the official line. Their first conclusion was that the Department of Health should make childhood immunisation a key performance indicator for Primary Care Trusts. (In other words, GPs should be given extra money if they met vaccination performance targets.) They also recommended that all London Primary Care Trusts `should appoint an immunisation champion to work with GP practices in order to boost immunisation rates'.

I could find no mention anywhere in the report of the existence of evidence suggesting that sticking needles and potentially dangerous substances into small children might not be a good thing. There was no discussion of the evidence that vaccines are dangerous and might cause serious damage to young children and infants.

Ironically, the title of the report was `Still Missing the Point?'

I rather think they are.

And I expect that at some time in the future the same merry group will launch an investigation into why the incidence of `autism' is increasing.

I began this essay by pointing out that these days doctors only get to hear and read what the drug industry wants them to hear.

It is not, of course, only doctors who are protected from the truth.

I haven't been invited (or allowed) to discuss vaccination on the radio or television for many years. This is largely because the medical establishment (having lost a long series of debates) will no longer agree to debate any medical topic with me or, indeed, to appear on any programme which has invited me to be a participant. (I have no doubt that an awful lot of untruths have been told about me by various representatives of the medical establishment.)

Not long ago, however, I was, to my immense surprise, invited to discuss vaccination on a late evening programme on Radio City, an independent station in Liverpool. A local doctor was invited to debate with me. The result was extraordinary.

For quite a while the doctor refused to admit that doctors make any money out of giving vaccines. Until I pressed him directly he indignantly denied that doctors have a financial interest in promoting vaccination. Only when I pointed out that GPs receive fees and bonuses for vaccinating their patients did he, rather reluctantly, agree that I was right. The doctor's main defence seemed to me to be that because the Government and other doctors agreed with his views on vaccination (which were, naturally, diametrically opposed to mine) then he must be right and I must be wrong. I have never found this a very convincing argument and nor, for a while at least, did the listeners. The presenter wanted to know why the facts I was giving had never been aired before.

At the end of the programme I was told that the programme had never before had such a response from listeners. It was, I was assured, their biggest ever audience response. Listeners were desperate for more information. Many were astounded at the evidence I produced. Some accused me of scaremongering for questioning pro-vaccination propaganda and for pointing out that doctors get paid for giving vaccinations. At the end of the programme I was asked if I would make another, longer programme on the subject of vaccination. I said I would. I offered to debate the subject of vaccination with any number of pro-vaccination doctors and experts the radio station could find.

I was not, however, surprised when I never heard from them again. I contacted them to ask if they were still interested in another more intensive debate. They weren't.

And since then no other radio station has been prepared to allow me to discuss vaccination on air. I doubt if this will change. Patients, like doctors, will be protected from the inconvenient truths.

The media in general is constantly full of articles and programmes sneering at those who worry about vaccination and promoting vaccination as safe and effective.

Here's an extract from a pro-vaccination article by a columnist in *Time* magazine: `I'm pretty confident in the way I get my knowledge. Even in the age of Google and Wikipedia we still receive almost all our information from our peers. When presented with doubts, I don't search for detailed information from my side. I go with the consensus of mainstream media, academia and the Government. Not because they are always right but because they're right far more often than not, and I have a TiVo to watch. Also, unlike anti-vaccination people, they usually shut up after a little while.'

I could hardly believe that when I first read it and I can hardly believe it now that I've re-read it. But the truth is that most people now think like this and so the bad guys get away with their lies and their deceits and their manipulations and their spin. The drug companies are extremely powerful and effective at persuading journalists. They have bought most of the doctors and most of the medical journals and so they can be very convincing. Sometimes the pro-vaccine journalists become quite absurdly overblown in their support for vaccination. In December 2009, a magazine called *Wired* even claimed it was a `fact' that: `By any measure of scientific consensus, there is total agreement: vaccines are safe, effective and necessary.' And it's a fact that the moon is made of green cheese. Facts? Who needs the real thing when you can just make them up when you need them.

Most doctors are unquestioning - too frightened to upset the establishment. Asking uncomfortable questions can ruin a doctor's career. And medical journalists are just as useless. Most have very little formal medical training, they don't know what to look for, they not infrequently receive payments from drug companies (the payments are offered for articles written for drug company publications and are frequently far in excess of the sort of payments that the journalists would normally expect to receive) and they hardly ever have the courage to take on the establishment.

Far too many so-called medical and health journalists are wimpy incompetents who won't print or broadcast anything which might damage their cosy relationships with the medical establishment and the international pharmaceutical industry.

The power of the pro-vaccination lobby is powerful and far spread. When I wrote a short-lived column for the *Oriental Morning Post* in China the editors were at first reluctant to publish a column I had written criticising vaccination. Eventually, the editors printed the piece (simply because I refused to provide an alternative). After the column appeared, my book publishers in China wrote to tell me that the Chinese Government had informed them that they could no longer publish my books. My publishers in China had produced four of my books, all of which had sold very well, but they had been told by the Government that only `medical publishing houses' could in future publish books concerned with health care. Other Chinese publishers who had shown great enthusiasm for publishing my books suddenly changed their minds.

I am sometimes told that, as a critic of vaccination, it is my job to prove that vaccines are dangerous and that I should stop criticising vaccination until I have evidence proving that vaccines can be dangerous and are often ineffective. That is a nonsense. It is the responsibility of those who are making, endorsing and giving vaccines to be sure that they are safe. The drug companies have a responsibility to prove that their products are safe and effective. Unfortunately, it is common these days for Governments to allow industries to do things without proving that they are safe, and to then expect opponents to prove that something is unsafe. The same thing happens, for example, with genetic engineering and genetically modified food. The fact is, of course, that it is impossible to produce evidence proving that a procedure doesn't do something. The onus should, of course, be on those who promote these procedures to produce evidence proving that they are safe. There is no evidence that genetically modified food is safe to eat because the people selling the stuff haven't done (or been expected to do) any research proving the safety of their product. Opponents and critics are dismissed airily and told that it is their responsibility to prove that genetically modified foods are unsafe. However, without vast sums of money, and access to the company's laboratories, that simply isn't possible.

In truth, of course, it is not the job of those who oppose vaccination to prove that it is not safe or effective. Indeed, even with unlimited resources it is nigh on impossible to prove a negative. How can I prove conclusively that the man down the road hasn't ever cheated on his taxes? How can I prove beyond any doubt that the Government hasn't ever tapped your telephone?

In a logical, sensible, scientific world it is the job of those who promote vaccination to prove that the procedure is safe and effective in general, and that individual vaccines are safe and effective in use.

Sadly, that isn't going to happen.

The problem (as the drug companies know only too well) is that when you start doing really serious research there is a real risk that you will obtain results that are commercially inconvenient. And the drug industry, the Government and the medical profession all have a vested interest in ensuring that vaccination programmes continue. If inconvenient truths were uncovered the drug industry would lose billions, the Government would find itself paying out billions in damages and individual doctors would lose thousands of pounds a year in lost fees and bonuses. So, there is no incentive for anyone to do any proper research.

Supporters of vaccination, who ignore this absence of evidence in their favour, have been conned by the establishment into believing that vaccines save lives. They are often abusive and sometimes almost hysterical in their attacks on the few doctors who dare speak out, and on those who dare to try to share the truth about vaccination with patients and with parents of young children. It is, perhaps, not surprising, therefore, that most doctors who worry about vaccines say little and do nothing in public.

However, readers may be interested to know that, contrary to popular opinion, a good many doctors *are* worried about the medical profession's unbridled enthusiasm for vaccination. Most (quite sensibly) prefer to remain anonymous.

Here is one (of many) relevant letters which I have received from practising doctors in recent years. This one came from a GP. He wrote: `Your criticism of vaccines is entirely justified. The medical profession has come under the baleful influence of the drug companies and so doctors have to pretend that vaccines can do no harm. I am a doctor and regard vaccination as a fraud and a farce. The witches in Macbeth might well have included modern vaccines in their recipe.'

All of us who criticise vaccination should take heart from American producer Jerry Weintraub, who once wrote: `If a bunch of men are discussing you, meeting about you, and scheming to destroy you, it probably means you're doing something right.'


# 28. Conclusion

The establishment always elevates its official beliefs into an orthodoxy; always suggesting that they are right because they are, well, right and that the absence of evidence is not to be allowed to interfere with the acceptance of their conclusions. This is tabloid science. And so, for example, the supporters of vaccination deal with opposition not by debate but by denouncing anyone who dares to question the orthodoxy or to murmur disagreement.

Back in the 1980s I dared to question the argument that AIDS would kill us all. Ignoring the available evidence as an inconvenient truth, the medical establishment had gravely announced that by the year 2000 we would all be touched by AIDS. It was official scare mongering. I was roundly attacked by the profession, the politicians and the media for questioning the logic of these claims and for daring to introduce embarrassingly accurate fact based arguments into the arena. No one in the establishment wanted facts which got in the way of their prejudices. I was (quite literally) banned from television for offering an alternative viewpoint and for daring to suggest that maybe AIDS might not kill us all after all.

It wasn't the first time I had been censored for daring to tell the truth. And it wasn't the last.

Today, the establishment has quietly forgotten its dire predictions about AIDS. New scares, often just as tenuous as that one, are presented almost weekly as researchers and drug companies fight for funding and profits.

It's the same approach as is used by climate change advocates. Critics who dare to question the establishment's fragile conclusions are demonised as flat-earthers or holocaust deniers, or accused of being in the pay of someone or other (although in truth all the money is on the other side of the debate). The only debate allowed is about the *size* of the problem we have created - we are never allowed to discuss whether climate change is man-made. Anyone who disagrees with the establishment viewpoint is dismissed as a dangerous heretic - to be excluded from all debates, and condemned and isolated. The blindly loyal flourish, thrive and enrich themselves; the honest purveyors of truth struggle in the dark.

Medical science has been hijacked by politically correct lobbyists. Dissenters, daring to question the new orthodoxy of the group-think obsessionals, are found guilty of thought crime and sentenced to be vilified and suppressed. Group-think unoriginality oppresses and suppresses. Vaccination is just one of many areas of medicine now considered to be beyond debate.

I believe that anyone who vaccinates a child should be arrested. I recognise that this isn't the official viewpoint. But why don't those who favour the official viewpoint (that vaccines are safe and essential) debate the issue? (Vaccination is by no means the only issue which is never debated in public. Other medical issues which are never debated openly include chemotherapy, radiotherapy, vivisection, drug therapy for the menopause and heart surgery.)

The modern medical establishment has made enormous and hugely devastating errors in recent years. The medical establishment was dangerously (and now provably) wrong about AIDS. The medical establishment was dangerously (and now provably) complacent about the dangers of overprescribing tranquillisers. For years the establishment ignored the link between tobacco and cancer. For years I was vilified whenever I argued that there was a link between stress and high blood pressure. The medical establishment still ignores the evidence proving that meat is the biggest killer in the so-called developed world. The medical establishment, which long ago sold out to any industry prepared to pay a decent price, always goes along with whatever is convenient and profitable and always opposes evidence which threatens the commercial status quo.

Today, more than at any time in history, medical schools teach half-truths; they never teach students how to think or criticise the system. (What system is going to teach people to question itself?). Students are educated by rote; taught in the way that dogs are taught tricks. Wisdom is a disadvantage. Common sense is eradicated. Young doctors are incapable of making informed decisions and that suits the pharmaceutical industry just fine.

But if you don't question perceived notions then how do you ever learn? How does a profession ever progress if no one is allowed to question the establishment's accepted beliefs? Young doctors are never exposed to the truth or to the questioning of `accepted' beliefs or to proper debate (e.g. with people like me). So medical schools churn out platoons of unquestioning, prescription-signing zombies. Originality is now a dirty word within the world of medicine. The establishment has deliberately and cold-bloodedly created an environment in which original thinkers are dismissed (by medical professionals, politicians and journalists) as nutters or fools who care nothing for the truth. Those who oppose vaccination are savaged as madmen who will happily see small children die in their millions.

Good doctors need insight, imagination and intuition and the capacity to make diagnostic leaps, sideways if necessary. They need to be able to observe and they need to be able to think if they are to serve their patients properly. But these skills are not simply discouraged; they are now not allowed. As a result the medical profession is packed with drudges; unthinking human dross, too frightened of losing their jobs to show any spirit.

Doctors do not have the courage to question the establishment or to have original ideas because they are employed by the State and like all other employees they are frightened of losing their jobs. Today's doctors are bought, body, mind and soul, and do not have the courage to stand up for whatever principles they might have had when they started out. They dare not disagree with their administrative bosses because they are hired hands. They dare not stick up for their patients because they live in fear of bureaucratic censure. And so they vaccinate, and they perform unnecessary operations and they prescribe drugs which they know are unsafe. Tonsils, breasts and lengths of intestine are ripped out by surgeons who don't have the foggiest notion of the harm they are doing. (And, seemingly, wouldn't give a damn if they did.)

Doctors do not have the courage to stand up for their patients because they have lost their independence; they are simply civil servants; they have sold their souls for a fat salary, short working hours and membership of a wonderful pension scheme. They are so beholden to their employers that they dare not even stand up to bullying, they dare not even speak out when they see things happening which they know, in their hearts, are wrong. Their spirits have curdled.

Medicine today has become rigid, like other forms of science, and original thinking is as unacceptable today as it was in the days when Semmelweiss was vilified. The medical establishment has never been enthusiastic about new ideas. After all, the medical establishment stoutly rejected anaesthesia and the principles of antisepsis and the brave physicians who promoted such ideas had to cope with rejection, cynicism and oppression. The doctors who have made the greatest contributions to health care have invariably been attacked, scorned and imprisoned. Things have not got better. Indeed, they are worse today than they have ever been. Today, anyone questioning the establishment is suppressed rather than just ignored. History shows that great and useful medical discoveries are invariably made by outsiders and mavericks; doctors and scientists operating outside the cosy world dominated and controlled by back-scratching establishment flunkeys. But in the past such outsiders did at least have a chance to make their contributions. They were reviled and ignored but (with surprisingly few exceptions) they were not silenced in the way that original thinkers are silenced today. The modern medical establishment was bought by the drug industry decades ago. Today, there is no room for initiative and originality and both are actively suppressed. Dissent is officially stifled. The great men of medicine, heroes such as Snow, Semmelweiss and Lister, would not have survived in today's environment. Anyone who studies medical history can see that the significant developments always come from free thinkers outside the system. Today, more than ever, the free thinkers outside the system are suppressed. They will doubtless be defrocked when the new rules of revalidation are introduced to protect the establishment and the pharmaceutical industry.

Traditionally, the medical establishment has quite a record of supporting the wrong view. Today, the power of the establishment to suppress makes things a thousand times worse. Existing therapies which are dangerous, ineffective and even lethal are protected. Antibiotics are wildly overprescribed. Benzodiazepines are still prescribed in massively dangerous quantities - creating millions of addicts. Patients are routinely dispatched to profitable screening clinics which do far more harm than good. Animals are slaughtered in laboratories which are used to preserve the profitability of the drug industry at the expense of patients. Vaccines are injected by the lorry load and children are paralysed and killed by the classroom.

Any doctor who disapproves of vaccination, or questions the effectiveness or safety of something that has become accepted as just as essential and as normal and as safe as food and water, is treated as a dangerous lunatic. Critics are silenced. Alternatives are not even considered. Eyes are closed to the dangers of genetic engineering and the reckless overprescribing of dangerous prescription drugs. The potential advantages of alternative remedies are dismissed out of hand simply because they might threaten the profitability of the industry which now owns what used to be a profession. As I explained in *How To Stop Your Doctor Killing You* it has been proven without doubt that most heart surgery is unnecessary. A sensible regime of diet, exercise and stress reduction can reverse the problems now regarded as indications for surgery. But the establishment continues to promote surgery because it is enormously profitable. New, innovative, safe and effective ways of dealing with diabetes are ignored, suppressed even, because they threaten corporate and professional profitability. Doctors don't bother looking at scientific evidence any more. It tends to get in the way of profits. The dangers of electricity, mobile telephones and prescription drug contaminated drinking water are all ignored because drawing attention to these threats may prove financially embarrassing to other parts of the establishment. Powerful evidence proving that all these are real health problems, responsible for many thousands of deaths a year, is suppressed without hesitation.

The medical establishment is nearly always wrong. It has always been nearly always wrong. And as pseudoscience develops and the drug company lobbyists push their patented cures faster and harder so they cause more and more problems.

Iconoclasts are never popular. The people who own and worship the icons don't much care for them being smashed. And these days the icon owners have all the power and most of the money. They control the politicians, the legislature and the media.

Just about every major advance in medicine has come as a result of the work of eccentric, passionate, determined unclubbables who have fought the establishment and who would today almost certainly fail the registration, licensing and revalidation procedures designed to ensure that only doctors who obey every rule of the establishment will be allowed to practice. Advantageous changes to society happen only through the determined work of unreasonable men. Great things happen only when enough unreasonable men care and are brave enough to be unreasonable in public. All real progress is made as a result of observation and deduction but these skills are not valued today. Just about all great discoveries in history have been made by people who weren't recognised by their peers before they made their discoveries and often weren't recognised for years afterwards either.

There has been woefully little really original thinking in medicine in recent years. This is partly because medical education discourages original thinking, the medical press suppresses original writing and the medical establishment outlaws original thinkers. It is, therefore, hardly surprising that there have been very few medical breakthroughs, no critical studies and hardly any bright ideas. Controversy is suppressed and the obvious ignored for fear of upsetting any part of the Unholy Trinity (doctors, drug companies and politicians) and of upsetting Government protected industries.

Over the last few years it has become increasingly clear that bankers, lawyers and politicians have all betrayed us. Despite my best efforts, the public has not yet realised that doctors have betrayed us too. And it will, perhaps, be some time before people realise that whereas politicians, lawyers and bankers have merely impoverished us, doctors have killed our relatives, our friends and our neighbours, have enriched themselves through their legalised slaughter and will most probably kill us too.

My theories of bodypower (described in my book *Bodypower* and to the annoyance of the medical establishment now proven to be accurate, sensible and economical) have been attacked and suppressed simply because they are accurate, sensible and economical. How can medical professionals make money out of a system which relies upon allowing the human body to protect and to heal itself? (Just the other day I read about a woman who had a baby which refused to take milk from her right breast. The baby would only take milk from the woman's left breast. The woman went to see her doctor who found a lump in the right breast. That's bodypower. But how can medical professionals make money out of that? And so, because there is no opportunity for profit, they sneer.)

The solutions modern doctors come up with, and the research results they produce are rarely original or creative or effective. They simply follow the party lines. The majority of today's researchers are simply messing around at various levels of unimaginative incompetence. They know that if they want to receive the best grants they must never question the effectiveness of the medical establishment and they must always worship at the shrine dedicated to the pharmaceutical industry.

When I was writing my book *The 100 Greatest Englishmen and Englishwomen* I was initially astonished at the number of great people who had spent at least part of their lives in prison. The explanation, of course, is that many great men and women, and almost all original thinkers, are, by their very nature, intrinsically rebellious and therefore especially likely to get into trouble with the authorities. And, after all, no one ever did great things by agreeing with the establishment; no one ever changed things for the better without having original ideas. And original ideas are always, almost by definition, an anathema to the establishment.

All great innovations, inventions, ideas and developments come from crazy, neurotic people. They may be a little bit or a hell of a lot crazy but they are all crazy. They may be odd but they certainly aren't boring, sensible or entirely stable. Great advances are never made by people who would be voted into office, made Head Girl or put in charge of the milk.

Things are set to become much worse.

New regulatory licensing schemes for doctors mean that practising doctors will have to be revalidated by a senior doctor who makes recommendations about a doctor's fitness to practise. It seems likely that this will mean that any doctor who does not stick to the rules will be refused a licence and prevented from practising. Just about every significant doctor in history, from Semmelweiss to Snow, would have failed the licensing scheme as planned and I have absolutely no doubt that the new system will ensure that any doctor who opposes, questions or in any way criticises vaccination will be removed from the medical register before you can say `scientific bigotry'. The chances of doctors questioning the medical establishment in the future will be close to non-existent. Today, money talks loudest and doctors listen to nothing else.

I have for many years been concerned about the safety and efficacy of specific vaccines. Those fears have gradually gelled into a general conviction that vaccination programmes are neither sufficiently safe nor sufficiently effective to be acceptable. And, of course, it is worth remembering that those involved in trying to `sell' vaccination programmes to the public have repeatedly lied and tried to prevent the publication of the truth. It is also worth remembering that those who promote vaccination usually have a good deal to gain financially, whereas those who oppose vaccination usually suffer severe financial hardship if they dare to make their views known. There is a desperate, burning need for research into the effectiveness and safety of vaccines but no such research will ever be done because the people who might authorise the work know only too well that the results are almost certain to be financially inconvenient.

I have been writing about medicine, and exposing hidden truths, for long enough to know that it is unlikely that politicians will take any notice of my views on vaccination. Nor is the medical establishment likely to change the way it does things.

And since my books are now widely banned I know that very few people will read this book.

But you've read it. And so now one more person now knows the truth. Share the truth with your friends and relatives. And, together, maybe we can change things.


`Strive to preserve your health; and in this you will the better succeed in proportion as you keep clear of the physicians.' - *Leonardo da Vinci*

# Postscript 1

You will probably have gathered, by now, that my view is that vaccines are unsafe and worthless. I would not allow myself to be vaccinated again. This is, however, a purely personal view and in fairness I stress that it is not a view shared by the majority of doctors, nurses, health visitors, journalists and war criminals. Readers must make their own judgements based on all the available evidence. I strongly recommend that anyone contemplating vaccination discuss the issue with their own medical adviser.

The bottom line is that I do not advise anyone not to be vaccinated, or not to have a child vaccinated because I am merely an author: it is not my job to tell people what to do. My role, as a writer, is merely to provide information (which isn't provided by the Government or the medical profession) and to give some idea of the sort of questions which readers may like to ask when considering a vaccination programme.

So, before you allow your doctor to vaccine your child (or you) you may like to ask her or him these essential questions:

1. How dangerous is the disease for which the vaccine is being given? (Exactly what are the chances that it will kill or cripple?)
2. How effective is the vaccine?
3. How dangerous is the vaccine? (Exactly what are the chances that it will kill or cripple?)
4. What side effects are associated with the vaccine?
5. Which patients should not be given the vaccine?
6. Will you guarantee that this vaccine will protect me (my child)? If not - exactly what protection will it offer?
7. Will you guarantee that this vaccine will not harm me (my child)? If not - exactly how risky is it?
8. Will you take full responsibility for any ill effects caused by this vaccine?
9. Is the vaccination essential?

Then ask him or her to sign a note confirming what he or she has told you. If your doctor or nurse wants to vaccinate you, ask him or her to confirm in writing that the vaccine is both essential and safe and that you are healthy enough to receive it. You may, I warn you, notice his or her enthusiasm for the vaccine (and your company) suddenly diminish. Ask your doctor or nurse to give you written confirmation that he or she has personally investigated the risk-benefit ratio of any vaccine they are recommending and that, having looked at all the evidence, they believe that the vaccine is safe and essential. How could any honest, caring, well-informed doctor or nurse object to signing such a confirmation - effectively, accepting responsibility if things go wrong?

Similarly, parents who are worried about having their children vaccinated should ask their doctor or nurse to sign a form taking legal responsibility for any adverse reaction. (Curiously, they might find doctors and nurses slightly reluctant to do this.)

It is important to remember that most of the doctors (including nearly all GPs) who write and speak in favour of vaccination are making money out of it. On the other hand, doctors who oppose, or even question, vaccination, do not stand to gain anything but are, on the contrary, putting their careers at risk.

Finally, ask the doctor to tell you the batch number of the vaccine. And keep the name of the doctor, the date and time and the batch number of the vaccine. And the surgery or clinic address. Lawsuits against doctors, drug companies and the Government usually fail because people don't have this information.

## Postscript 2

A few years ago I wrote a book called *Coleman's Laws*. Here is Coleman's 8th Law Of Medicine: `The medical establishment will always take decisions on health matters which benefit industry, Government and the medical profession, rather than patients. And the Government will always take decisions on health matters which benefit the State rather than individual patients. What you read, hear or see about medicine and health matters will have more to do with the requirements of the pharmaceutical industry and the Government, than the genuine needs of patients.'

## For a full list of books by Vernon Coleman please visit http://www.vernoncoleman.com/

Printed in Poland
by Amazon Fulfillment
Poland Sp. z o.o., Wrocław